Mother Nature s Diet

Mother Nature's Diet

Lose weight and feel great

By Karl Whitfield

MND Health Ltd
Mother Nature's Diet - Lose weight and feel great. Second edition
By Karl Whitfield

ISBN 9781795439060

Contents

Introduction

D iets are rubbish! Most of the time, they don't work! You will be relieved to know that *Mother Nature's Diet* is not 'just another miserable diet'. It's a healthy lifestyle. Let me give you some quick reassurance by explaining the difference:

- No starving, no suffering
- No calorie counting
- No fad behaviour
- No **temporary** 'give up this', or 'eat that'
- No 'guilt trip' language – you don't have to confess your sins, count your 'bad points' or report your weight every week

That's the stuff of fad diets, and research proves that fad diets generally don't work[1]. In most cases, people lose a few pounds on the temporary diet, but then put it back on again as soon as they revert back to old habits. That's not what *Mother Nature's Diet* is all about. Instead, we use the word 'diet' in its correct meaning.

> Diet, noun
> 1. The kinds of food that a person, animal, or community habitually eats.
> 2. In nutrition, diet is the sum of food consumed by a person.

This is how we use the word diet in this book, rather than the fad diet meaning of "Stopping all your bad habits for a while, losing a few pounds in time for that beach holiday, then going back to your old behaviour and wondering why

---

[1] *Dieting does not work, UCLA researchers report.* April, 2007. http://newsroom.ucla.edu/releases/Dieting-Does-Not-Work-UCLA-Researchers-7832

you put the weight back on again!" Fad diets regularly don't work for the majority of people, for two main reasons.

Firstly, the behaviour pattern of the diet is not sustainable, so eventually the 'diet' ends and the person reverts back to their old ways. As they go back to eating what they used to eat and doing what they used to do, they typically regain most of the weight they lost – often all of it, and more! This applies to all those silly fad diets, where you starve yourself on some low-calorie regime, eating nothing but cabbage soup and apples for weeks on end, or something equally unsustainable like that.

Secondly, the person fails to stick to 'the diet' plan. This is very common, the old 'falling off the wagon' problem. This often happens because the plan or dietary regime is too miserable, restrictive or arduous to follow. Or because the person is 'in the wrong place' mentally and emotionally, they lack the right mindset and the right motivation, or perhaps they lack support – at home and work.

Three things to learn

While you read this book, as well as introducing you to the *Mother Nature's Diet* healthy lifestyle, I hope to teach you three things.

1. You have a choice. The value of preventive medicine.
2. Eat less, eat better, move more.
3. You are an individual. One size does not fit all, we are all different. Aim for progress, not perfection. Healthy living doesn't need to be hard. You *can* do it, just start.

Along with a host of tips and useful information, it is my hope that you will learn these three simple but important lessons while reading this book.

What is Mother Nature's Diet?

Mother Nature's Diet is a healthy lifestyle. It's a way of living, including dietary guidelines, to help you lose unwanted weight, have plenty of energy, avoid ill health and resist the signs of ageing as best as possible. *Mother Nature's Diet* (or 'MND' as many followers like to call it) is designed to help you feel great, look your best and enjoy your life in every way.

Mother Nature's Diet is a complete, balanced healthy lifestyle, covering diet, exercise and lifestyle. The *Mother Nature's Diet* lifestyle offers you the best way to eat and to live for:

- Good health
- Abundant natural energy
- Longevity – we want to live for a long time, but we want those years to be productive, healthy years. It's not just about lifespan, but 'healthspan'. *Mother Nature's Diet* is about adding years to your life *and* life to your years

However, it's not **only** about *you*. We also connect human nutrition with the natural world, the environment and agriculture. We are interested in the best way to create a sustainable future, where we all eat for good health, but where we also improve animal welfare for farm animals and minimise the impact of agriculture on the environment. Eating the MND way is also designed to help:

- Reduce greenhouse gas emissions
- Sustainably manage ocean fish stocks
- Reduce atmospheric pollution
- Encourage sustainable topsoil management
- Stop the destruction of rainforests
- Minimise the desertification of grasslands

In the long term, *Mother Nature's Diet* is an abundant healthy lifestyle designed to promote ways to feed us *sustainably*, helping to promote good health for *all* – humans, animals farmed and wild, the land, the oceans, the air and all living things.

Personal responsibility

Mother Nature's Diet is for people who care, people who want the best for themselves, and people who are prepared to put in a little effort to get permanent lasting results. *Mother Nature's Diet* is all about taking personal responsibility, and working on yourself to get the best out of your life, in every way.

There is certainly an element of *personal development* involved, this lifestyle is about being the best version of you that you can be. Whether you are currently aged 30 or 70, if you are the kind of person who refuses to accept that turning 40 means "it's all downhill from here" and if you believe that we can be slim and healthy and full of energy in our 40s, 50s, 60s and beyond, then the *Mother Nature's Diet* way of living just might be the lifestyle you have been searching for.

If you think the right way to live is to eat fresh whole foods, rather than searching for answers in the form of supplements, pills and powders, then *Mother Nature's Diet* will resonate with you.

"Doc, can't I just have the pills?"

A while ago I interviewed an NHS GP about the state of healthcare in the UK, and I asked the questions 'Are people working hard to help themselves?', and 'Do most GPs prescribe drugs too easily, without promoting healthy lifestyle advice?' I was told, and I was shocked, that while many GPs do take the time to give lifestyle and dietary advice, repeatedly, the reality is that a staggering *nine out of ten patients* just disregard that advice and ask "Doc, can't I just have the pills?" This is the sad truth – the NHS is going bust because people are not taking personal responsibility. Nine out of ten people. That is shocking and saddening to me.

If you just read that little story and, in your mind, you thought "I'm the one in ten, I don't want to just take pills, if there is a way that I can help myself, then I will." If that's you, then you'll find that *Mother Nature's Diet* is the lifestyle for you. You will enjoy this book. *Mother Nature's Diet* is the meeting point of personal development and lifestyle medicine.

If you want to lose that excess weight for good, no more fad diets, no more yo-yo weight loss, then *Mother Nature's Diet* may be the answer you have been looking for. If you are prepared to get outside every day for some fresh air, take long walks at the weekends and switch off that TV from time to time, then you'll feel right at home living the MND way. If you want more energy, and freedom from sugar-lows and the afternoon slump, then MND just might be for you.

What is Mother Nature's Diet not?

This is not just 'drop a dress size in time for the holidays!' *Mother Nature's Diet* is not just a weight loss program, it's not just a quest for a 6-pack and it's not a 'muscle building program'. MND is not a sports nutrition plan, to help you lift heavier, cycle faster or run for greater distances, however, it will help you to be healthy on the inside, which should aid you in whatever sports or exercise goals you pursue. If you want to lift heavier, run faster or cycle further, this healthy way of living should help you reach those goals – it certainly has helped me to do all those things!

> *Mother Nature's Diet is not a fad diet! This is a long-term lifestyle, not a short term quick-fix!*

MND is designed to help you be the best, healthiest version of you possible, healthy on the inside, looking good from the outside, feeling healthy, energetic and confident, to help you achieve whatever life goals you have. MND is about living longer – we want to add years to your life, **and** life to your years. *Mother Nature's Diet* is the place where preventive medicine meets personal development. The best version of you: fit, healthy, and full of energy, now and far into your future.

Our goal, our mission

The mission of *Mother Nature's Diet* is to inspire and help as many people as possible to find the best natural way to achieve supreme good health and abundant energy. *Mother Nature's Diet* started out as my own personal mission to transform my own health, but as people became interested in what I was doing, and the beneficial results I was getting, it has grown.

The following definition, give or take a few words, was the original goal I set out to achieve for myself, and this now has become the *Mother Nature's Diet* definition of supreme good health and abundant energy. This remains my own personal goal, and I hope it can be a goal you strive for too.

- Free from pain, disease, immobility and any obvious illness
- Abundant vibrant energy
- Resisting the signs of premature ageing – maintain youthful looks and energy levels
- A good level of basic fitness, strength and flexibility
- As a minimum, moderate physical ability across a range of functions
- Attractiveness – clear skin, not too fat, not too thin, bright healthy looks, a fit sexy body (however you define that, what makes you feel happy and self-confident)
- Natural virile healthy sexual function and high libido
- Longevity – the ability to live a long, healthy life, free from disease and disability
- Age well – maintaining excellent levels of physical and mental ability well into old age
- Happiness

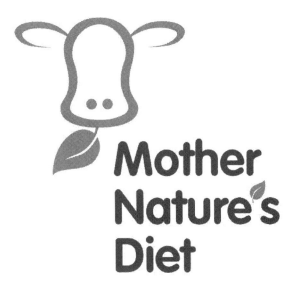

Our founder

Mother Nature's Diet was started by me, Karl Whitfield, in 2011, borne out of a combination of my passion for healthy living, my own personal health transformation and my frustration with the endless confusion and complexity that pervades the worlds of weight loss, health and nutrition.

I fought with excess weight for over 20 years, yo-yo dieting in and out of obesity for two decades. I smoked for 20 years, and was a heavy drinker for 26 years, and suffered a variety of minor health complaints. Then, between my mid-30s and mid-40s, I turned that all around, lost over 100 pounds of unwanted fat and became a picture of health and fitness. You can read more about my story in the next chapter.

The 12 Core Principles of Mother Nature's Diet

Mother Nature's Diet is made up of 12 Core Principles, a simple set of guidelines about how to live, eat and move your body. These are 12 simple points to guide you to optimal good health. The 12 Core Principles are easy to understand, easy to implement and easy to follow. This book is your introduction to the 12 Core Principles of *Mother Nature's Diet*. You can visit my site at *Mother Nature's Diet* (dotcom) any time to print off copies of the 12 Core Principles to stick to your fridge or kitchen cupboards or anywhere else that it helps you. Just visit www.mothernaturesdiet.com/12-cp

See image overleaf.

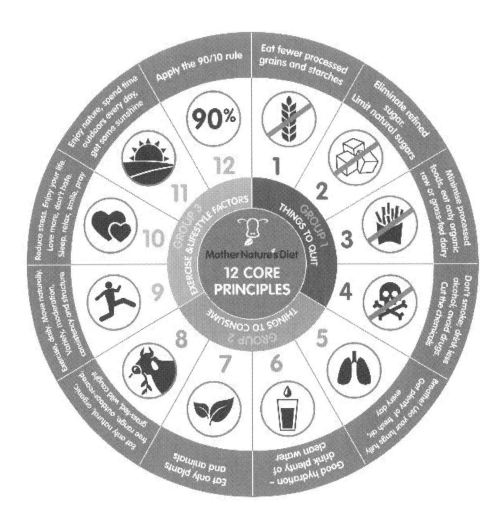

My Story

"WHO THE HECK IS THIS GUY AND WHY SHOULD ANYONE WANT TO LISTEN TO WHAT HE HAS TO SAY?"

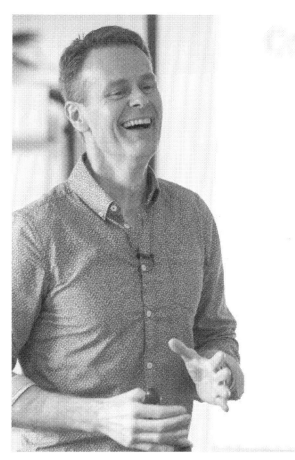

Image credit: Craig Fletcher Photography
London, January 2017, with thanks

I am not a doctor, not a qualified Dietitian or Nutritional Therapist, I don't have a PhD in biochemistry and I am not employed as a cancer research scientist or any such thing. Understandably, this may lead you to ask the question – just who the heck is this Whitfield bloke and where does he get his information from, and why should I believe a word he says?

Great question. The short answer, in two sentences, would be this.

I'm just a 100% regular guy, I was 'getting it all wrong' health wise for 20 years, smoking, drinking far too much, yo-yo dieting in and out of obesity, I had health problems, took prescription medications for 17 years and I was overweight, out of shape, unfit and unhappy. That was 20 years of my life. I know how that feels.

Then, between my mid-30s and mid-40s, I turned it all around, quit my unhealthy addictions, lost 101 pounds (46 kilos or 7 stone 3) of unwanted body fat, got fit and ran a bunch of marathons, cured my health problems and sorted my life out; all while reading 847 books and research studies along the way to become something of a walking encyclopaedia of health and nutrition knowledge. All tried and tested on myself.

That's the short version, skipping on a lot of detail, that's as short as I can get it. So, rather than being highly qualified academically, I feel I am qualified in 'been there, done that' real-world **experience**. I am not anti-science, anti-academics, anti-doctors or anti-medicine. To be clear, I hate all that pseudo-science nonsense as much as anyone, it drives me crazy. I believe in evidence-based medicine, I think our fantastic NHS is a world-class service and I am vehemently opposed to bits of it being sold off and privatised, and I 100% support all the wonderful doctors, nurses and specialists who train for years and work so hard to provide the incredible service that they do.

You will not read one word of 'anti-medicine' mumbo-jumbo in this book, and you will never hear me putting down our health professionals. I despise all that ludicrous conspiracy theory crap about 'the truth about this and that' and 'what the doctors don't want you to know' and 'they are keeping you sick for profits' and so on. I refuse to waste my time with such garbage. I don't believe in magic pills, I don't believe some superfood from a Tibetan mountain is going to save us all, and I can't stand snake oil salesmen any more than you can.

But while I fully believe in evidence-based medicine, I also appreciate that there is a role for anecdotal and experiential evidence. My own life experience, my own health transformation, explained in detail below, has taught me far more than all the books and studies I have ever read. Nothing in a book can teach you what it's like to be overweight and obese for 20 years and then work your tail off to lose over 100 pounds of fat. No book can teach you how it really feels to have chronic low self-esteem. No research study can give you that feeling. Real life is not a controlled study. Real life is not a text book.

So far, science just does not have all the answers. Some things take many, many years to reach scientific conclusions. And some studies will never be done, it's just not possible. This is particularly true of studies that track the long-term effects of diet and lifestyle choices and how they affect us over a period of many decades.

Imagine, if you will, the recruitment process for this research study…

"Wanted, 600 parents to please sign-up your new born children to 80-year experiment. 300 will be fed a perfect healthy diet of organic veggies, grass-fed meats, sustainably-caught wild fish, they'll be kept from smoking and drinking for ever, they will be given a low-stress life, good hydration, and plenty of sleep. The other 300 will be fed crap and made to start smoking as teenagers, we'll get them pissed up five nights per week for most of their adult lives and stress them out daily. We'll deprive them of fresh air, exercise and sunlight, and we'll ensure they are vitamin D deficient, they'll never eat their 5-a-day and we'll make them work long hours on night shift, sitting down, on saggy uncomfortable chairs, working with hazardous chemicals without proper safety equipment. Let's see who dies young. Please apply in writing to…"

We good? Yeah, you parents, are you up for it, shall we get you guys and your new-born babies signed up for this project?

Noooo!! Of course not!! Right! Some studies just can never be done, they are impossible, unethical, impractical, too time consuming and too expensive, for all manner of reasons. So, the evidence base of scientific research that we do have available to us is limited to what we can study, to what variables can be controlled, and to the time scales that researchers can work within, based on practicalities such as funding and study attrition rates.

For many reasons it might take decades to find answers to complex issues, such as the percentage of the population who might suffer some kind of gluten intolerance, and is it really the gluten, or is it the FODMAPs, or is it the glyphosate (pesticide) sprayed on gluten-containing staple crops? We might not know, for sure, 100%, for **decades yet**. Meanwhile, while we await a *firm answer from science*, I could find 50,000 people who will tell you, anecdotally, that when they eat bread and pasta, they get gastrointestinal bloating, noisy farts, and they tend to gain weight. When they cut out the bread and pasta, the symptoms go and they lose weight.

The evidence is anecdotal, and there are many scientists online suggesting that the jury is still out on gluten. But if you are 45 years of age, 30+ pounds overweight, you tend to feel bloated after eating certain meals, and you get gas in the afternoons and evenings, wouldn't you want to try 90 days without gluten-containing starchy carbs to find out if that's the cause of your problems? That's where *Mother Nature's Diet* Core Principle 1 comes in, and the ethos behind the 12 Core Principles: try it. Try 90 days off the cereals, breads and pasta, try it and see. If it makes no difference, you lose no weight and you feel no better, then fine, throw out MND and keep looking for the answer that works for you. But I can tell you, I've been doing this for a decade and so far, and I can promise you than 99% of people I meet, benefit from cutting back on those starchy carbs.

> *"To be crystal clear, I don't have an academic degree in anything. I have a 'life degree' in losing 101 pounds of fat and getting my shit together."*

I may not have a PhD in biochemistry, but the 12 Core Principles of *Mother Nature's Diet* are based on everything I learned over the last 30 years, and the many hundreds of books and studies I have read. The advice in this book is simple and mainly based on common sense, and my invitation to you is this: **just try it and see how it works for you**. If it doesn't help you, you've lost nothing. No expensive supplements, no promise-laden superfoods, no complex calorie counting. Just simple common-sense healthy living.

I'm not a medical doctor nor a PhD and I don't pretend to be. I'm just a regular guy, I'm like you, I struggled with excess weight and feeling less than my best for years. And then I beat it all, I turned my health and life around. **If I can do it, so can you.**

To be crystal clear, I don't have an academic degree in anything. I have a 'life degree' in losing 101 pounds of fat and getting my shit together. That's the best thing I have to offer. I was going to stop there and claim that's the sum total of my qualifications, but for what it's worth, I am actually a qualified Personal Trainer too, and I guess that counts for something - at least I am qualified to give you exercise advice and nutritional advice for activity.

Legal medical disclaimer

I'm not a medical doctor, nor a qualified State Registered Dietitian, nor a Nutritional Therapist, nor am I a scientist, I do not work in research labs, and I am not employed in the pharmaceutical industry. I'm not a medical student, nurse, surgeon or oncologist, nor am I in any way qualified to give anyone medical advice.

I am not a doctor; I am not pretending to be; I am not trying to be.

The F Word

For many years of my life, I was a fat guy. Woah! I used the 'F' word! "Oooh, he said 'fat' – doesn't he know that's not politically correct these days?!?!"

I'm sorry, I say it like it is, please don't be offended. I do not say 'fat' to offend anyone, it's not a slight on your character, it's not an attack on your personality, it's just a description that we all understand and all relate to. Know that being overweight, being obese, being 'fat' is just a particular arrangement of molecules in your body. It's not permanent, it can be changed, it doesn't mean you are ugly, it doesn't mean nobody loves you, it doesn't mean you're not good enough, it doesn't mean you're a horrible person and it doesn't mean you are any less of a person than anyone else. It's just an arrangement of bodily tissues.

But let's not mess around with any of this 'person of a larger build' or 'big boned' or 'it runs in my family' stuff. Let's just be honest about where we are at – and if we are not happy, and it's harming our self-esteem, and if we accept that obesity is unhealthy, then let's do something about it. So, I use the F word occasionally, it's no big deal. You know, I have the right to say fat, because I've been there, I've done it. I was that guy. That was 20 years of my life.

And I then lost 101 pounds of fat, that's 7 stone 3, or 46 kilos if you speak European. I spent 20 years doing the whole yo-yo dieting thing, fat years and thin years, up and down on that roller coaster. I tried all kinds of crazy fad diets. I did all the wrong things for my health. I smoked for 21 years. I was a pretty heavy drinker for about 26 years, and I had a fairly unhealthy relationship with alcohol, lacking much self-control, I liked to drink pretty much every day. I knew nothing about diet until I was around 35 years of age. I lived on bagels and peanut butter, sliced white bread, milk, red wine, beer, cheese and cigarettes. I didn't know how to cook vegetables, I didn't really know what to do with vegetables. I thought salad was boring.

I went through periods of using exercise as a weight loss tool, and long periods as a TV addict.

From the age of 17 onwards I suffered from an undefined type of nasal rhinitis. I lived every day of my life feeling like it was the first day of a heavy cold. My nose poured day and night, eyes itchy, sneezing and sore throat, permanently bunged up. I went to my doctor as a teenager, two doctors actually, and they said they didn't know what was wrong with me. I was given a prescription steroid nasal spray and told to use it twice daily for the rest of my life - at 17 years old. After taking that stuff for 18 years, I cleaned up my diet and lifestyle, and the condition went away.

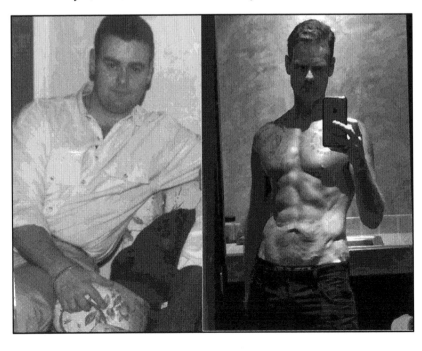

In my early 30s, I became an urticaria sufferer. When I was run down, or when my skin got cold, the skin all around my mid-section, arms, wrists, fingers, legs and bum would erupt in angry, red, hives all over these areas. It would flare up quickly and I'd be stuck with it for weeks at a time, even months in a single stretch, itching day and night. It would often be accompanied by something called angioedema, where my lips and parts of my face would swell up, and my tongue would swell up inside my mouth, to several times its regular size, filling my mouth.

I'd be worried I was going to fall asleep at night and I'd stop breathing or something. I had all these things wrong with me, the urticaria, and the angioedema, the nasal rhinitis, and the doctors had no idea why, so they put me on prescription steroidal antihistamines. These strong antihistamines would whack me out, I would be so drowsy I couldn't stay awake to drive a car, I would be so drowsy I was slurring my words as if I was drunk. I'd fall asleep reading to my kids or sat at my desk working. I took these drugs for about seven years, the doctors just said 'take them' for however many years I needed to. Yet, I cleaned up my diet and lifestyle, and it all went away.

At the age of 35, I had a bit of an 'epiphany moment' when we had our first baby, and I kind of looked down at this kid in my arms and I thought… "do you know what? I'm heading in the wrong direction. I'm on the wrong path, here, this isn't how I want to live my life."

I don't have many 'before' photographs from my teens and 20s, because they hadn't invented digital cameras and mobile phones back then, and as a fat bloke lacking any self-confidence, I was pretty camera shy. If any friends or family members did take pictures of me, I tended to hunt them down and destroy them…the pictures that is, not the friends and family! While avoiding cameras, avoiding ever being seen in public with my shirt off, and avoiding mirrors whenever possible, as I progressed into my 30s, I had this nagging though that occupied my mind…

"I could see my future self, a costly NHS statistic in-the-making"

There I was in my early- to mid-30s, I had just become a father for the first time and just started my own business for the first time, and I realised I was heading in the wrong direction. I was heading along a road that, to my eyes in that sort-of-epiphany-moment, looked like I was very likely setting myself up for:

- Obese, unfit and sedentary in my 30s (I was already there)
- Type-2 diabetes in my mid-40s (like so many people I meet, especially men)
- Classic candidate for heart disease in my 50s (obese, smoker, diabetic, high blood pressure, poor diet, heavy drinker, sedentary, all markers for heart disease)
- Likely dead from cancer in my late 60s (a fate that has befallen several in my family; hardly anyone on my mother's side reached 70 years of age)

This is not what I wanted from my life!!! I looked at my little baby (well, not so little actually, he weighed over 10 pounds at birth, so he was a big baby really) in my arms, and I thought to myself "I really want to live to see this guy grow up, and get married, and get a job, start a business, have his own children, stuff like that. I want to live a long time, and feel good, and have energy to enjoy my children and my life."

I realised that I needed to change direction in life, before I became one of these statistics that we hear about that's crippling the NHS, dealing with this chronic disease burden. I could see my future self, a costly NHS statistic in-the-making, and I decided it was time to change.

Somewhere around my 35th birthday I reached a point where I had had enough. I had yo-yoed back up to 240 pounds/110 kilos/17 stones and I was smoking again (I quit a thousand times…some lasted a month, some lasted a few hours) and I decided I had to change. What was different this time to every other time before, was a change in mindset. Previously, I had always thought things like…

*"I **should** stop smoking, it's bad for me, and it causes cancer."*

"I really want to lose some weight so I don't feel so embarrassed out in public."

*"I **shouldn't** drink so much; it's such a waste of money."*

But these thoughts never carried much 'emotional weight' in my mind, I don't know why but they just didn't inspire me or motivate me. But this time was different. This time I had been asked the question "Who are you? Who do you want to be? What is your identity?" and in a flash I answered "I want to be a healthy person, one of those fit, bubbly, energetic, wholesome, earthy-types, strong and vibrant. I want to be healthy." And it was like 'Boom!!' and fireworks were going off in my head!

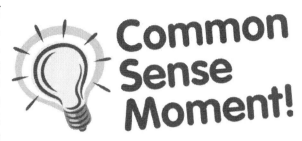

Common Sense Moment!

I know that sounds cliché and cheesy, but it was all unplanned and unexpected, that's just how it happened, that was my lightbulb moment! I stood up, walked to the nearest bin, took out my packet of cigarettes, scrunched them up in my hand and threw the mashed-mess in the bin. Previously, I would always "stop at the end of this packet" or "today is my last day" but this time was different, this time I just threw them away and have literally never wanted one since, not for over 13 years now. In my mind, I was a healthy person, and healthy people don't smoke. I had changed my identity, and quitting smoking was instantly effortless.

From that day forward, I started to learn about being healthy. I stopped 'trying to lose weight' and just focussed on being a healthy person. Excess body fat fell away almost effortlessly, I quickly lost the first three stones in just a few months. I started to exercise every day, I started to cook and eat vegetables, salads, fresh fruits. I massively reduced my alcohol consumption and drank more water, and everything changed.

Over the next few years, I lost 101 pounds of fat, that's 46 kilos or 7 stone 3 in 'old English'. I have never smoked again, I quit drinking completely, and I got super fit. I got into running and completed a dozen marathons, a couple of ultramarathons, and cycled from John O'Groats to Land's End. I ran a PB marathon of 3 hours 14 minutes aged 40, pretty good going for an ex-20-year-smoker. I learned to love doing push-ups, and once did 2500 in five hours.

The rhinitis, urticaria and angioedema all went away, I stopped the medications and was soon in the healthiest, fittest state of my life. I've faced a few hiccups along the way – the running became a bit obsessive and I ended up in knee surgery. I had an accident when I was 42 that left me with a double-fractured spine. I fell off the side of a mountain when I was 44 and slid 250 feet down an ice field, and stopped by crashing into a wall of ice using my chest as a brake. That cost me five broken ribs.

But all these injuries have healed fast, something else I put down to being in great health. In every case I have taken no medications, very few painkillers, and just kept moving gently and shunned rest, and I seem to heal with amazing speed.

In my early 40s I became a qualified Personal Trainer, and I became obsessed with reading books about nutrition, diet, heart disease, fitness, cancer, training, running, weight training, diabetes, nutrients, disease, anything to do with health and wellbeing. Over the last 13 years I have read over 847 books, research papers and studies, covering all these topics and more. And I have spent many thousands of pounds of my own money attending courses, seminars, training events, lectures and conferences to learn about every aspect of health, nutrition and disease prevention.

Reading all those books and research papers, one thing that used to drive me absolutely nuts (and still does) was the mass of conflicting information, the endless contradiction, where literally none of these experts can ever agree with each other!

You read this one book, written by some highly-qualified PhD 'Dr this' or 'Dr that', and it's all backed up with 38 pages of references at the back, all those little super-script numbers in the text telling you where the information has come from, it all looks very legitimate and scientific, it reads well, is articulate, intelligent, logical, and seems to be extremely believable. Then you read the next book, written by an equally well-qualified 'Dr such-and-such' and with a comparable slew of references, and all looking equally scientific and well written and believable...and it draws completely the opposite conclusion!

Aaaarrrggghhhh!!!! Who to believe?!! I was a complete novice, just a regular layman, just some guy who spent 20 years fat and drinking and smoking, I left school when I was 15 years old and no one in my family ever went to university, we weren't 'that sort of family'. How the heck was anyone supposed to make sense of all this!

- Don't eat dairy, it's 'cow puss' that will fill you with mucus and give you breast cancer and autoimmune disease!
- Dairy is the original 'superfood'! Go dairy crazy, it's packed with nutrients and great for building muscle!
- Healthy people don't drink coffee
- Coffee is a great healthy natural stimulant, perfect for athletes!
- Go Paleo – caveman just ate meat all day, so we should eat loads of meat
- Don't eat red meat, it gives you heart disease and bowel cancer!
- Saturated fat is bad for you

- Saturated fat is good for you! It's the sugar that is bad for you!
- Sugar is good for you, it gives you energy!!
- Your diet should be 55% starchy carbs. Grains and cereals and bread and pasta, these foods should form the bulk of your diet and they give you all your energy
- Go ultra-low-carb, it's the starchy carbs making everyone fat!
- Eat low-fat foods for weight loss
- Eat a low-carb, high-fat diet, it's the best way to lose weight!
- Avoid meat and fatty foods so you can bring down your cholesterol, because high cholesterol causes heart disease
- Screw cholesterol levels, cholesterol is good for you, so stop worrying about it
- Vegetarians are healthier and they live longer
- Vegetarians don't live longer, it just feels like it!
- Vegetarians only live longer because they tend to smoke and drink less
- Alcohol is killing you
- Moderate alcohol drinking is better for you than not drinking at all!
- Do lots of running and swimming and cycling to burn off fat
- Cardio will trash your joints! Stop running and lift weights
- Weights are best for burning fat
- Eat more protein to build muscle
- Don't eat too much protein, it's bad for your organs

SSSSTTTTTTOOOPPPPP!!!!!
Aaaaarrrggghhhh I can't cope!!!

I read loads of books and went to loads of seminars, I watched a ton of videos and webinars and started trying to make sense of these research papers, and it all just got so confusing, I had no idea what was the right thing to do. So, I became my own test subject. I would pick a book, follow the plan or advice, try it on myself for 30 days or 6 months or whatever seemed appropriate, then keep a record of the results. And repeat. Again, and again.

I bought supplements, gadgets, superfoods, exercise equipment. I tried fad diets. I gave up whole food groups. I went vegetarian. I ate meat until it was coming out of my ears. I drank milk, I quit milk. I ran. I lifted weights. I went low carb. I went high carb. I tried it all. I spent (erm, wasted) money on pendants to keep unwanted electromagnetic frequencies at bay. I bought a water ionizer for over a thousand quid. I tried green drinks, alkaline water drops (quack nonsense!), muscle building BCAAs, creatine monohydrate and protein powders.

I read everything.
I tried everything.

Surviving the madness

From age 35 to 45 I put myself through all that, and what came out the other end was me, 101 pounds of fat lighter, 20 odd pounds of muscle heavier, fit as a fiddle and the healthiest I have ever been in my adult life. Out of all of it, what worked? From the fancy supplements, the over-priced superfoods, and the expensive kitchen gadgets, what actually got the results? Well, what came out was *Mother Nature's Diet* and the 12 Core Principles.

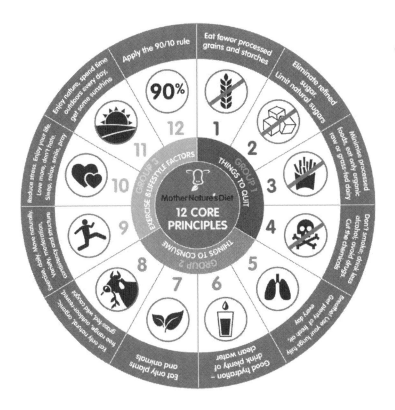

Personally, I think 99% of the supplements, superfoods, kitchen gadgets, expensive pieces of home workout kit and all those endless 'diet books' are all a total waste of your time and money. I am sure some of that stuff works some of the time for some people, but none of it did much for me, and I haven't met many other people for whom some superfood or supplement was the secret to their success. For most people, common sense healthy living, and some discipline and hard work, gets the best results.

I believe that pretty much all you need to know, for most people to get the results they are after, in terms of losing weight, shaping up, feeling great and doing the best you can to hold back the signs of ageing and prevent the onset of degenerative disease, is all in this book you are reading right now. It's all in the 12 Core Principles of *Mother Nature's Diet*.

- Eat a diet comprised mainly of fresh whole foods
- Don't smoke
- Drink less alcohol
- Keep away from refined sugar
- Exercise often, daily is best
- Stay active
- Consistency is king
- Sleep more, reduce stress, chill out
- Drink plenty of water
- Get some fresh air and sunshine
- Enjoy some variety in your exercise
- Buy organic
- Meditate, take time out, time away, offline, in silence

I went from being this low energy, fat, drunk bloke with a cigarette in his mouth, to being this lean, fit lively guy who never runs out of energy. I never get sick. I never get coughs or colds, and my chronic health conditions went away. 18 years of prescriptions went away. The doctors told me they didn't know what was wrong. Now I know: I was unhealthy, I was living out of whack with the natural world, with Nature, with the biochemical processes that go on inside my body a million times a day.

I learned to look after myself, I healed myself, I got fit and lean and healthy. I learned to analyse the science to find the research which wasn't biased, to make sense of those research papers and diet books.

> *I went from fat, confused, medicated, drunk and low in self-confidence, to the best shape of my life - fit and full of energy, slim and strong, vibrant and healthy, and the nuts and bolts of everything I learned along the way are in this book. It's all simple common-sense, all laid out in easy-to-follow steps for you.*

I have been working with people over the last five years, helping folks to lose weight, have more energy and enjoy better health. In my experience, the most common reasons people give for not finding the time or energy to exercise, or for not cooking proper meals from scratch using fresh ingredients, usually include:

- I don't have time to exercise
- I have a demanding career
- I run my own company/am self-employed
- I have young kids/busy family life
- I'm too tired all the time
- We have a baby, so I don't have the energy, I'm too tired
- I don't know what to do/how to exercise/how to cook/what to eat
- I can't afford all that gym wear and the gym fees
- I can't afford to buy organic
- I'm too busy
- I'm too old
- I don't know where to start

I know how it is; *I have faced every one of those challenges myself* at some time. But the thing is, I made my health transformation between 35 and 45 years of age, while facing most of the challenges on that list. My wife and I had our three kids while I was between age 34 and 40, the same period of time when I achieved the bulk of my 101-pound weight loss. I was a very hands-on dad, doing my share of night feeds, pacing the room with a crying baby, early mornings, all that. Far from using the tiredness caused by the babies as an excuse that made healthy living harder...on the contrary, healthy living made coping with the tiredness from the babies easier.

It was also the same years (age 33 to 46) that I built and ran my own company and grew my career massively, often working 12 to 15 hours per day. I did it all at the same time. Again, far from the demands of my career making it harder to find time for healthy living – exercise, cooking and sleep. On the contrary, making time for exercise, cooking fresh nourishing meals and getting more sleep, helped me grow my business and function better in my career.

A decade ago, I was too busy, I didn't know what to do, I was too tired, I was confused, I had a demanding life, but I did it all anyway, I made the time, and soon felt the benefits.

If I can do it, anyone can do it: and that means you can do it too.

Approximately 14 pages back, I told you the short version of my story in just two sentences. (Phew, sorry the long version took 14 pages!!) Then I said I would tell you the long version to help you decide if you want to listen to what I have to say or not. Have I answered this question for you?

"Who the heck is this guy and why should anyone want to listen to what he has to say?"

- I'm just a regular guy, I have no special training, qualifications or advantage. I was not born to doctor parents, a rich family, genetically gifted, nor raised an aspiring young athlete
- I was heading along the wrong track, for over 20 years, in and out of obesity, on medications for minor chronic conditions, out of shape, unfit, lacking self-confidence
- I changed it all, lost 101 pounds of fat and got super healthy and super fit
- I have spat, pee'd, pooped and bled into pots and tubes and sent it all to labs for testing! I seem to be as fit and healthy as can be, inside and out
- I am not qualified to give you medical advice; I am not trying to supplant your doctor
- I only want to give you health advice, to help you be, and stay, fit and healthy
- I am a qualified Personal Trainer, I can legally give you advice about exercise and nutrition for physical activity

- I have read 847 books and research papers on every aspect of health, nutrition and disease
- I was not some genetically-gifted muscle-bound hunk at 22 years of age, looking perfect and feeling great. I was the obese drunk at 18, who yo-yoed until I was 35. **You're not too old**, it's not too late, you can change
- I made my change while exhausted from sleep deprivation and while building my business. No excuses
- If I can do it, **YOU** can do it too

The Lifestyle

So far you have read a fairly short introduction to this book, and then a rather long version of my story. Up to this point, I have already explained that –

- *Mother Nature's Diet*, or MND, is not 'a diet'! It is certainly not a 'fad diet' – it's a permanent way to life, a sustainable healthy lifestyle
- There is no fad diet behaviour – no calorie counting, no tracking your macros, no sin points to declare or any such thing
- I hate pseudoscience and quackery and snake oil sales scams as much as you do!
- I love science, I love evidence-based medicine, but I also value the role of anecdotal evidence and life experience. Real people trying to lose weight in the real world, can experience life quite differently to the controlled environment of a study
- In this book, you won't read a bad word said against the NHS, against doctors, nurses, surgeons, oncologists or any other healthcare professional
- I think the NHS only has one fault, one major problem, and it's not a lack of funding. The NHS simply has too many customers
- *Mother Nature's Diet* is not 'alternative medicine', it's **preventive medicine** – at MND, we want to help the NHS by lightening their load of future customers. We want to help **you** to not become one of those future customers
- MND is for everyone; everyone who is prepared to **take some personal responsibility** for their own body shape and their own future health outcomes. Because of that 'personal responsibility' thing, that means that 90% of people probably won't read the rest of this book and won't stick to the MND lifestyle. That's a sad shame, but that's just how it is. **I urge you to be in the 10%**
- MND can help you lose unwanted weight, get fitter, have more energy, feel great and improve your foundations of good health, for

- sport and training. MND can help you resist the signs of ageing and resist ill health as much as is realistically possible
- MND is about being the best version of you that you can be, with supreme good health and abundant natural energy as the foundations of all that you do
- This book is your introduction to the MND lifestyle and explains the 12 Core Principles to you in enough detail for you to get started and enjoy the immediate benefits
- This book includes a 28-Day Plan for you to follow. You'll need to tweak a few details to suit you as an individual, but the plan should be enough to get you started, to point you in the right direction

Most places I go, *most* people I meet, want to lose a few pounds. We certainly all want to look our best. We want to feel our best, healthy, energetic, self-confident, and look our best. Seriously, I have never met anyone who actually *wants* to look or feel like crap. We want to resist the signs of ageing. We want to look good for 30, good for 40, good for 50, good for 60, whatever age we are. I mean, seriously, no one wants to wake up in the morning, look in the bathroom mirror and think "Oh dear God I look bloody awful for my age, what a mess!" Nobody actually *wants* to think that. Right?

And I believe we all want to feel our best. We want to wake up in the morning vibrant, full of energy, feeling full of beans. And we all want to resist ill health, especially as we get older.

More energy

I truly believe we all want to look our best, and I think we all want to feel our best too. I think most people would like to have more energy. There's a great guy called Tony Robbins, who does personal development seminars and home-study self-improvement course. I once heard Tony Robbins in an interview, and he was asked the question, 'if you could do one thing that would have more impact than anything else on every area of your life, what would it be?' Without hesitation he answered "Have twice as much energy." Just think what it would do for your life if you had twice as much energy.

Think what it would do for your career prospects if you showed up at work every day with twice as much energy. Maybe you run your own business. Think what you could achieve in your business, and how you could improve sales and motivate your staff, if you showed up with twice as much energy at your business every day. Just think what it would do for your relationships, if you had twice as much energy to engage with your loved ones every day. Your spouse. Your children. Your friends, co-workers and customers. Think how much more you could get done in your life, more fun, more travel, more sex, more sport, more of everything you enjoy, it could all improve if you had twice as much energy.

I believe that every area of your life gets better when you deliver more energy to what you're doing. I also believe that our modern lifestyles and poor diets are not helping us to have abundant natural energy. Too many folks are eating junk food, not exercising enough, staring at screens too much, not getting much fresh air and sunshine and are chronically sleep deprived.

I believe that the *Mother Nature's Diet* lifestyle can turn all that around, and – like it did for me – you can go from being sick and tired of feeling sick and tired, to having abundant natural energy, never feeling ill, never taking time off sick, and getting much more done in your life. If you could stop feeling so tired, have more energy, and not keep losing five to ten days each year to minor illnesses, just think how much your life might improve.

Recently, I read (I think it was in a PwC report) that UK businesses, predominantly small businesses, are losing £29 billion per year because the average employee calls in sick for 9.1 days per year. That's pretty much two weeks, per person, per year. If you run a business, your staff are each calling in sick for two weeks every year. That's a huge business loss to minor ill health complaints and 'Monday-itis' that a lot of people seem to suffer from. And I read some government statistics for the UK economy as a whole over 2010, '11, '12, and '13, and for each of those four years, the UK economy as a whole, lost over £100 billion in productivity from people being sick, each year. Over £100 billion per year lost from our national economy because people are tired, sick, run down, suffering from mostly minor or preventable illnesses and feeling like crap.

We need to be healthier. People say they want to 'save the NHS' and I agree – and I think the best way to save the NHS is to take some personal responsibility for our own health, and do all we can not to become NHS 'customers' in the first place.

You have a choice

OK, this is probably the 'heaviest' thing I am going to hit you with in this whole book. Let's get this sorted early on, then everything gets easier from here on out!

You have more choice in your health outcomes than you realise.

This is one really big thing that I want to share with you in this book. You can exert more control than you probably currently imagine over these areas of your health: how you look, how you feel, how much energy you have, the size and shape of your body, your weight, your ability to resist the signs of ageing, your ability to resist ill health, and I'm talking about coughs and colds, and things like that. I'm also talking about more serious ill health, like cancer and heart disease, and autoimmune conditions, and type-2 diabetes, and more. *I believe you can control these things more than you probably know, more than you have been led to believe.*

You have a choice. But in my opinion, **a lot of people don't realise this**. I am sorry, this topic is rather morbid, but we need to talk about disease and death. Over the years, the things that kill us have changed. 20,000 years ago, our caveman ancestors were killed by predators, accidents and infectious diseases. High infant mortality was almost certainly the #1 cause of death for the human race. Then for a long time, in more recent history, it was wars, poverty, infectious diseases and malnutrition that were killing us. But through technology, medicine and public sanitation, many of those causes of mortality have been sorted out. Now, what kills most humans is NCDs, non-communicable diseases.

Non-communicable diseases

'Non-communicable' means they are not infectious, we don't 'catch' them, they 'develop' inside us. Worldwide, around 55 to 60 million people die every year. These NCDs account for about 70% of those deaths. The four things that kill most people are heart disease and stroke (circulatory diseases), cancers, diabetes and lung conditions.

What these diseases all have in common, is that they develop inside us, over time. **Another word for 'develop' might be 'grow'.** They *grow* inside us, and *therefore we have some opportunity and ability to exert an influence over that growth process.*

Of course, some of these diseases are unavoidable. Some people are born with heart problems, some people inherit a genetic 'malfunction' that can lead to a cancer forming at a young age, and some people inherit genes that make them predisposed to certain cancers. But in all, inherited conditions and genetic abnormalities only really account for about 10% or 20% of cancers, and less than 10% of heart disease. What of the other 80%? Well, we can exert some influence over that.

For instance, the #1 preventable cause of cancer worldwide is **smoking**. Smoking causes heart disease, lung cancer, other cancers and several lung diseases. According to WHO, the World Health Organisation, smoking is the primary cause of death behind roughly 10% of all human death every year. So, there **we have a choice**: don't smoke, and you should live a little longer.

See how this works?
You have a choice.

According to Cancer Research UK, the NHS, and other leading charities, approximately 42% of cancer deaths in the UK are caused by **smoking, obesity, drinking alcohol, poor diet, lack of exercise, irresponsible sun exposure** and exposure to **toxic chemicals** and similar hazards at work.[1] [2] [3]

Well, you can *choose* not to smoke, you can *choose* to eat sensibly, the *Mother Nature's Diet* way, you can *choose* not to drink alcohol, or to drink much less, you can *choose* to eat a better diet, more than your 5-a-day, you can *choose* to exercise regularly, you can *choose* to be sensible in the sun, and you can *choose* not to work in an environment where you may be exposed to toxic chemicals.

Just those things, in that last paragraph, that's **almost half** of UK heart disease and cancer deaths taken care of right there. You can *choose* not to be a part of that statistic. Just take a few moments to **read back over** the last few

---

[1] Brown, K., et al. (2018). The fraction of cancer attributable to modifiable risk factors in England, Wales, Scotland, Northern Ireland, and the United Kingdom in 2015. *British Journal of Cancer*, 118, 1130-1141. Retrieved from https://www.nature.com/articles/s41416-018-0029-6

[2] Cancer Research UK. *Cancer risk statistics.* (Various 2014-2018). Current estimates at https://www.cancerresearchuk.org/health-professional/cancer-statistics/risk#heading-One

[3] *Lifestyle changes could slash cancer rates.* (2011, Dec 7). Retrieved Feb 19, 2019, from https://www.nhs.uk/news/cancer/lifestyle-changes-could-slash-cancer-rates/

lines again, and really let that sink in. Go on, I encourage you, flip the page back and read it again, maybe a few times, really take it on board.

Now of course, let's *not* talk about **saving lives**. We *can't* save lives, we can only prolong them. Personally, I'm all for a longer life! The truth is, we're all going to die, one day, that's a fact of life. But average life expectancy in the UK is around 80, so I am saying you can choose, or at least 'stack the deck in your favour', do you want to go at 65, or make it to 95? How you live, I believe, can make that difference.

Many of the things that cause cancer, are the same things that cause heart disease. And it just so happens they are also the same things that cause diabetes (type-2) and certain lung diseases. While smoking is the leading cause of lung cancer, it is also the leading cause of COPD (chronic obstructive pulmonary disease) and it is one of the most well-established leading causes of heart disease.

Poor diet and a lack of exercise are the leading causes of obesity and type-2 diabetes. Obesity in turn is a major cause of heart disease and a direct cause of ten different types of cancer, including breast cancer and bowel cancer (all quoted from Cancer Research UK, with thanks). Being diagnosed with diabetes takes nine to ten years off your life expectancy, and diabetes in turn is a leading risk factor for heart disease.

You see, it's the same things, time and again, causing so much of our ill health. In this book, my message is simple...

You have a choice.

But the trouble is, I find a lot of people just don't realise it.
You can't choose, if you don't know.

Not-so-common knowledge

We grow up with 'common knowledge' like "Smoking gives you cancer" and "Being massively obese, you're a heart attack waiting to happen." and "My mum always said we should eat our fruit and veg." but beyond that, I find that most people really don't realise that if we all just made some smarter choices, we could hold off 50% of deaths in the UK for an extra decade or two, just through some simple healthy living. And heaven knows how this would ease the burden on our beloved NHS. And of course, beyond the UK, this is all broadly the same for most of other Western nations too. So, now you **do know**, that you have a choice. The question is, what are you going to do differently?

One size does not fit all

Human health is a complex topic. The body and all the systems and processes going on inside, and everything that causes those systems and processes to fail, to malfunction and breakdown, is all really very complex. It is all multi-faceted, or multifactorial, and in most cases, the causes of health problems are unique to the individual. We are all different, in our genetics, our microbiome, our inherited traits and our unique environment and situation, and it is combinations of these factors that lead to health problems.

Yet amid all this complexity, *so many people are looking for simple answers*. We **buy** simplicity, we **want** the quick fix, we buy the **pills and promises** of the diet industry, the supplement sellers, and the snake oil salesmen. Health and disease isn't that simple...*but we really wish it was!*

Get over it!

Embrace complexity. You don't have to become a PhD in biochemistry, but accept that the causes of heart disease and cancer and obesity are complex and technical and you cannot just buy some powdered Himalayan yak testicle, sprinkle it on your breakfast daily and you'll live to 104 and never get sick! That's a fairy tale!

We live in a society where so-called newspapers fill pages with pictures of celebrities and socialites, writing 'news stories' of where these people eat their dinner or crash their cars. These newspapers like to run news that sells, they like to print sensationalism and fear, because that's what sells papers. Reporting of health news and health studies in these newspapers is poor, simplistic and often exaggerated.

If a study follows 1000 people eating meat four times per week for ten years, and 1000 people eating no meat for the same ten years, and if three people die of colon cancer in the meat eating group, and only two people die of colon cancer in the vegetarian group, the study results go out saying that the *relative* risk of colon cancer for people eating meat regularly is 50% higher than for vegetarians. Because three is 50% higher than two.

A sceptic might say that at just two or three people in 1000, there is virtually no difference and the data is inconclusive. A scientist would understand that many other factors may have impacted on the results, and a scientist would dig in to the methodologies behind the study to see what factors were controlled for.

But among the general population, few people are interested in taking the time and trouble to understand complex things like 'what causes cancer' and to look at all those possible factors and variables. Most people want simple. And newspapers like to give it to them, with headlines like "Eating meat increases colon cancer risk by 50%." In reality, few people read beyond the headline and the first few paragraphs.

This allows the media to 'educate' us and this gives them a powerful influence in the decisions we make and how we live our lives. *The media are not to be trusted with this power!* They are not in business to guide your health decisions; they are in business to make money, for themselves and their shareholders.

We're all **playing the victim** when it comes to our health, and too few take the time to read and understand the complex causes of ill health. As I have explained in this chapter, you have more choice over your health outcomes that you have been led to believe, and there are things we can do during our lifetimes to minimize risk and help ourselves.

> *"Everything will work for someone, but nothing will work for everyone."*

I have recently been reading a lot of diet books and blogs and looking at some of the most popular diet programs currently in vogue. Within the space of just a few days:

- I read an excellent report on the benefits of ketogenic diets for type-2 diabetics and people suffering from neurodegenerative disease. The article was written by someone knowledgeable, intelligent, published and well-respected, and backed up by plenty of examples of people who have enjoyed success with ketogenic diets (personally, I know several people who get great results!)
- Then, without looking for it, the very next day I happened across a well-reasoned argument against ketogenic diets, again written by a knowledgeable trainer with a long track record of client success stories. He warned of the dangers of low carb diets negatively affecting thyroid function, and he shared many anecdotal stories of female clients who have suffered hormone disruption through

trying ketogenic diets. He also argued convincingly that ketogenic diets can cause some people to suffer sleep abnormalities, hormone problems, mood swings, anxiety and misery (life without carbs – not much fun!)

- Ummm, one blog full of reports of people going super low-carb and finally ditching that stubborn belly fat they wanted to get rid of. The other blog full of reports of people feeling tired, run-down, burnt out on ultra-low-carb, who then ate more carbs and felt strong again and saw that stubborn belly fat finally melt away! Confusion much!

- Then I was reading a book about the benefits of intermittent fasting and the health benefits of fasting in general. Again, a well-researched and well written book, lots of scientific references and plenty of anecdotal references too. Mental benefits, fat burning benefits, metabolic benefits, weight loss, improvements in blood sugar management, insulin sensitivity and more

- I had a look around online and found many blogs and groups proclaiming the benefits of intermittent fasting diets, full of weight-loss success stories...and I found a similar number of blogs and groups bemoaning that 'intermittent fasting diets don't work' or that as soon as they returned to eating normally, these people regained any weight they had lost

- I read a wonderful book a couple of weeks ago about some of the newest research into the effectiveness of Paleo diets and how many people enjoy weight loss results on a Paleo-style dietary regime. Then I read a series of very confusing blogs, and it became clear to me just how muddled the Paleo message has become. Some people seem to interpret Paleo as meaning 'fairly low carb', and some seem to think it means LCHF (low carb, high fat) and some seem to eat lots of carbs. Some think ketogenic diets are an extension of Paleo, while others look at hunter-gatherer tribes eating high carb diets (many roots and tubers) and argue that Paleo is actually pretty high carb

Oh, the glorious confusion! I found stories of folks getting weight loss results and improved health from all variants of this Paleo interpretation! These people were all following variations of what they believe to be a Paleo diet, some very low in carbs, some really quite high in carbs, and all achieving weight loss results. Then I searched around and found opposing legions of people complaining Paleo is too hard, Paleo is too restrictive, Paleo doesn't work and they failed to lose weight on a Paleo diet!

Now let's just see –

- Intermittent fasting – some people lost weight, some didn't!
- Ketogenic diets – work for some people, not for others!
- Paleo diets – some people get results, some people don't!
- Low-carb, high fat – works for some, not for others!

Well whaddya know, it's the same old story with diets that we have seen for decades – works for some, not for others. **Just maybe**, it's **not** the diet, maybe *it's the people!*

We are all different!

The truth is, *we* are *all* different. 100,000 people could go buy a diet book and 30,000 might find it works wonders, and 30,000 might find it fails badly and makes them feel dreadful or gain weight, and 40,000 might report 'no change', but that's because the people are all different and **no single diet works for everyone!** (Actually, if 100,000 people buy a diet book, the chances are 50,000 will never read beyond the end of the first chapter. But that's another story for another day.)

- Some people thrive on carbs, some don't
- Some people are highly active, some are not
- Some people thrive on a high fat diet, some don't. Some people have genetic variations that help them metabolise certain types of carbs, or certain types of fats, but others don't have those variations
- Some people have gut bacteria that suits digesting certain carbs or certain fats, others have a different bacterial make up
- Some people's genotype or phenotype suits a certain diet, some people suit another
- Some people are stressed to the hilt, others live a relaxing life. Our stress levels affect our hormones, which in turn affect our digestion, metabolic function, weight and body composition, among other things
- Some people live in so-called 'obesogenic environments' while others live and work in healthier, more natural environments

All these factors (and many more!) determine how your genes, your gut, your blood, your metabolism, your muscle mass, your endocrine system, your sleep patterns and your lifestyle will interact with your diet. **It's no wonder 'one size diet does not fit all' when you realise how very different we all are.**

And that's why I often say that the 12 Core Principles of *Mother Nature's Diet* are guidelines, sign posts to help you navigate your way to find the perfect diet for you.

The 12 Core Principles are, I believe, the best all-round health advice I can offer to a nation wallowing in obesity and non-communicable degenerative disease. Given that *we are all different*, and given that the perfect healthy diet for anyone **is the healthy diet they stick to**, these 12 simple one-liners, in the plainest English possible, make a solid starting foundation for most people. But they are **not** a one-size-fits-all prescription. That's just *not possible*. You need to try these Core Principles out, and find the ones that work for you as an individual.

For one person, the 'cut the grains and starches' advice of Core Principle 1 may be perfect, but another person may do better keeping a few starchy potatoes and some organic oats in their diet for extra energy. Another person may be entirely gluten-tolerant and thrive with a little sourdough bread as their weekend treat.

For one person the 'no alcohol' advice of Core Principle 4 may be the best health advice they ever received, but for another person, the stress-relieving benefits of a glass or two of red wine once or twice per week may make for a healthier life balance in the long term.

One person may interpret Core Principle 12, the 90/10 Rule, as 75/25, and another person may thrive on 95/05 – maybe it all comes down to age, genetics or lifestyle pressure!

> We each have to find the perfect diet for us. I offer the 12 Core Principles as a framework, broad general guidelines, purposefully open and non-prescriptive, a baseline to help you find the perfect healthy diet for you.

What did we learn in this chapter?

You took some time to think about what it would do for your life if you had twice as much energy:

- Your career
- Your love life
- Your sex life
- Your bank balance
- Your family life
- Your sports and hobbies
- Your sense of wellbeing
- Your self-esteem and self-confidence

I introduced you to the idea of *preventive medicine*. **You have a choice.**

- I truly think that most people are not aware that a huge percentage of the chronic disease burden in our society is largely preventable, through better diet and lifestyle choices

One size does not fit all. We are *all* different, and the only perfect diet *is the diet you stick to*, for life.

- If it's heinous and you can't make it stick then it's clearly not a sustainable healthy way to life long-term
- Our goal is to be healthy and maintain a healthy weight – this should not mean suffering some ghastly regime, starving and feeling awful

Everything will work for someone, but nothing will work for everyone – remember that when you are looking at testimonials for the diets you see promoted online and in books and magazines. Can you see, those three things I said I was hoping to share with you in this book (on Page 2), those lessons are starting to come through now?

It's time to look at the 12 Core Principles now. It's time to see how you can lose weight, have more energy, improve your health, hold back the signs of ageing and be the best version of you possible, all by following the MND lifestyle. **So, go on then, let's get cracking.**

The 12 Core Principles

When I was 18 years old, with a huge belly hanging over my trousers and smoking two or three packs a day, I used to work in a print and bookbinding factory. It was a hot summer (this would have been 1988) and I worked on the end of a folding machine. Sections of books were printed up 16 pages to a sheet, then this machine folded them up so that all the pages fell in the right place, up the right way, in the right order. The machine spat out the sections of folded-up pages in great fistfuls, every few seconds.

My job was to stand on the end of this machine and catch these folded sections in big batches as they came out and stack them on a pallet, to go off and be bound into complete books. On this particular day, as the machine cranked away, I was sweating to keep up with it – it never took much to get me sweating, when I was a 250-pound lard-arse. One of my nicknames in those days was 'lard'.

I wore a scruffy beard back in those days. As the sweat poured down my face, it 'funnelled' through the beard and came out the end in a steady drip. I looked down at one point and realised that the drips, as they dripped out of my beard, were landing on my belly, creating a large wet sweat patch on the front of my shirt. I pressed the pause button on the machine and looked down at my belly for a few minutes. I let this image sink in.

After my shift finished, a couple of hours later, I went home and stripped down to my boxer shorts. I stood and looked at myself in the mirror for a while. I tried a set of push-ups, and as memory recalls I managed about eight or nine. I tried some sit-ups and if I remember correctly, I only managed a few before squirming and giving up at the effort. I went back to the mirror and took stock of where I was at in my life. This 'young man in his prime' at 18 years of age.

I was sure I had read or heard somewhere that a man's testosterone production peaks at around 18. Age 18 is the peak of muscle-bound manliness, and then it's downhill all the way from there. I was sure I knew that. I looked at myself, stood there in just a pair of boxers, and that was the first day I decided I had to change, I had to sort my shit out. I was a mess.

I knew nothing back then about disease or healthy living. If you had said to me that I should stop smoking or drink less because it might kill me, I would have shrugged (in my 18 years of worldly wisdom) and said 'good, who cares'. It's hard to motivate someone to look after themselves and stop the self-destructive behaviour when they have chronic low self-esteem, they wallow regularly in self-loathing and they think 40 years of age is ancient and to live that long would only prolong the misery anyway.

No, my brain thought nothing that day of being healthy. I just wanted to lose some weight so I might look a bit more attractive, in the **hopes I might get laid a bit more often!** Ah the mind of a young male!! What a deep and complex well of psychological wonders it can be!

Sex and beer! My world!

And so began the yo-yo years, the fad diets, the attempts to lose weight. Fast forward 27 years to my mid-40s, and the end result is the 12 Core Principles of *Mother Nature's Diet*, representing the distilled wisdom of my learning over 16 years of doing all the wrong things, and 11 years of getting it right.

As we work through the 12 Core Principles over the coming pages, I will give you **weight loss tips, anti-ageing tips, cancer-prevention tips, heart disease prevention tips** and more. I will help you learn how to **have more energy**, look and feel your best and **resist ill health** as much as is realistically possible. Then we will summarise some of the points in easy bullet-point lists at the end, quick summaries you might like to copy out and put up somewhere, maybe in your kitchen.

You are going to have to change

I'll be the first to agree, that change can be hard. But you have to understand something important - if you keep doing what you've been doing, you'll keep getting what you've been getting.

If you keep doing what you've been doing, you'll keep getting what you've been getting.

If the 'results' in life you've been getting are fat, weary, feeling and looking like a sack of shit, lacking self-confidence, unhappy with yourself, how you look and fell, then I think it's time to change the 'doing' side of the equation. Don't you?

The MND lifestyle that I promote ***does*** require some additional effort...you have to shop in different places, spend your food budget differently, make time to exercise, spend a little extra time cooking. It is all an effort and I can understand that in many circumstances, it takes people some time (or perhaps they just need the **right** time) to face change.

My advice would be...

...just start.

Don't be sitting around waiting for the right moment, don't pursue perfection, don't get wrapped up in planning and preparation...

...just start.

I mean, you've carried that extra weight for years, right? You've faced those low self-confidence feelings for years, right? You've avoided cameras, mirrors and tight-fitting clothes for years, right? So frankly, the best time to start might have been years ago, right? Well then, let's not waste another moment. There's no time like the present. Let's just get cracking. With all that crap behind you, why delay any longer...?

...just start.

What's involved?

You'll be glad to know the 12 Core Principles are really pretty straight forward and easy to follow, they are quite user friendly. *Mother Nature's Diet* is all just simple, common sense advice. It's not rocket science, you don't need a PhD to understand it, you don't need to spend £300 per month on supplements and superfoods, and you don't need to keep a detailed food diary every day. There is no calorie counting, tracking your macros, starving yourself, eating ice cubes or developing any kind of eating disorder!

The premise behind *Mother Nature's Diet* is simple – "Follow these 12 simple ideas, consistently, for life, and you will enjoy the best health possible, maintain a healthy body weight, do your best to protect yourself from chronic disease and you can get on with a normal life without feeling like you are living under some strict, detailed dietary regimen."

These are 12 simple points to guide you to optimal good health. The 12 Core Principles are easy to understand, easy to implement in your life and easy to follow. Living this way requires no science degree, in fact, it's quite the opposite. I have worked hard to remove the science and complexity, and the end result is purposefully simple, as good health should be. And far from starving, this lifestyle is abundant, you shouldn't need to suffer in order to be healthy.

Giving people dietary advice in the 21st century has become a dangerous game, fraught with complications and **whatever I say, someone will criticize it, contradict it or say that it's wrong.** The reality is that all dietary advice is open to variation - all people are different, your metabolism is different to someone else's, your gut flora is different to someone else's, how you absorb and assimilate food is different to someone else. The mineral content of food varies according to the soil it was grown in, the geographic location, the climate, the season, the environment. The amount of exercise and activity you do which you define as "an active lifestyle" may be very different to someone else's definition. One person is an athlete, the next person is not. One person wants to lose weight, another wants to gain weight. Many factors are involved, we are all different.

Across all this diversity, the 12 Core Principles are designed to create the best possible outcome for the broadest population possible. I believe the 12 Core Principles are an excellent, healthy, optimal and abundant way to live for the overwhelming majority of people, but of course, some people may disagree. I am sure it would be impossible to prescribe any one lifestyle for all people, everywhere, that would work for everyone. That's just not realistic.

I suggest you try the 12 Core Principles, treat them as guidelines rather than 'hard rules' and see what works for you. Strictly regimented eating rules tend to be a hallmark of the fad diet world. Instead, the 12 Core Principles are a broad set of basic guidelines that work **most of the time for most people**. I encourage you to try them, and *adopt what works for you*. Adopting a healthier lifestyle long term is more about finding what works for you as an individual than about following the latest predetermined set plan just because it happens to be endorsed by some celebrity!

If you would like to print off a copy of the 12 Core Principles to use at home or in your office, you can visit the webpage https://www.mothernaturesdiet.com/12-cp to download an image of the 12 Core Principles to keep and print and share with friends. Maybe it will help you to put a copy up in your kitchen at home, and one at work too!

Remember...

- You are going to have to make some changes
- Those changes are probably going to feel uncomfortable at first
- Hang in there, you'll soon get used to it

> **If you keep doing what you've been doing,**
> **you'll keep getting what you've been getting.**

- Just start
- The 12 Core Principles are basic guidelines
- They'll help you find the perfect diet for you. The perfect diet for you is the one that you stick to and you get results

Great, it's time to get going...

...just start.

You can use this page for your own notes.

Core Principle 1

I n today's diet-obsessed world, carbohydrate (carbs) consumption has become one of the most over-discussed and hotly-contested issues in modern day nutrition, and it is all-too-easy to get lost in the detail of the arguments. However, this book is not the place for that, so I am keeping this necessarily brief.

Mother Nature's Diet is not a strict low-carb diet as has become very popular in recent years. While there is no doubt that low-carb and ketogenic diets (ultra-low carbs) have proven to be extremely beneficial for some people, that is not what we are advocating here. Living the MND way, carbs are on the menu every day – vegetables and fruits are natural carbs. We eat 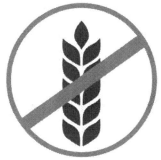 vegetables at pretty much every meal, and fruits in moderation. Beware of diet advice that eliminates entire food groups, such as "don't eat carbs" as this is often a sign of nutrition advice that is restrictive, trying to apply 'one size fits all' mentality where it does not suit everyone.

In very broad general terms, there are five key reasons why we avoid eating processed grains and starchy carbs when living the *Mother Nature's Diet* way.

1. For the vast majority of people, unless you are an athlete, you just don't need lots of bulky starchy carbs in your diet. The truth for most people is that eating lots of these starches provides a lot of carbohydrate calories you just don't need, and that can lead to a gain in excess body fat.

2. Grains cannot be digested unless they are processed or fermented, and in the natural order of things, way back in our evolution, these foods would not have formed a major component of our diet.

3. Most of these foods (grains) naturally contain compounds that are not good for a lot of people. These foods contain gluten, phytic acid and other chemical compounds that can cause digestive problems.

4. Grains and starchy carbs – the way they are consumed in the typical Western diet – tend to supply lots of bulk and lots of calories, without supplying much in the way of micronutrients – vitamins and minerals. **In terms of eating foods that fill your plate, there are much better choices.**

5. Modern large-scale industrialised agriculture, particularly grains and other staple crops (including wheat, corn, rice, barley, sugar and soybeans) agriculture, is a major source of topsoil erosion and greenhouse gas emissions.

This book does not allow us the space to explore each of these points in great detail, for that you might like to visit my blog or keep an eye out for my future books, so here we will just touch on these topics very briefly. Mainly, we are looking at points 1 and 4 from above, to keep things simple and brief.

Your bread is making you fat

Eating lots of processed carbohydrates and starches – **that's bread, pancakes, cereals, pastry, pasta, white potatoes, spaghetti and rice** – can contribute to gaining excess unwanted bodyfat. In very plain English: too many starchy carbs can make you fat.

The 12 Core Principles of *Mother Nature's Diet* are an attempt to give the best possible nutrition and lifestyle advice to the broadest possible group of people. In the world of nutrition, one size never fits all, so there will always be people who will disagree with Core Principle 1, but we believe this advice stands true for 'most' folks eating a typical Western diet. Athletes with specific training goals and individualised energy requirements would be the major exception.

It's important to remember:

- One size does not fit all
- I'm not saying "everyone should quit bread, it's bad for you"
- But...bread isn't what it used to be!
- Bread used to be known as 'the staff of life' but bread has changed. Nutritionally, there is a world of difference between a hand-made organic, fermented, sourdough loaf, and a typical UK-supermarket loaf of sliced white

- Broadly speaking, for most people, too much bread, cereals, pasta, rice and so on is adding lots of additional carbohydrate (sugar) calories to their diet, and leading to weight gain

It's all the excess carbohydrate in our diet that is exacerbating this worrying obesity epidemic that we are witnessing. Additionally, there is considerable evidence suggesting that it's contributing to the prevalence of type-2 diabetes too. Since the end of the 1970s our government has been telling people to base a third or more of their diet on these starchy carbs, these so-called 'slow burn' or 'slow release' complex carbohydrates.

The trouble is, over time, the nation has taken to eating huge amounts of these breakfast cereals, and all this white bread and white pasta and rice, at the same time as becoming ever-more sedentary. Statistics show that only around 30% of women and 40% of men in the UK even manage the government's minimum recommended amount of weekly exercise, and that target is set pretty low. Our kids are taught at school that we need 'slow burn' carbs for energy, and these foods should form the base of our diet, but the problem now is that folks are eating a ton of carbs then sitting on their butt all day and not burning it off!

Buns, bagels, baguettes and big-bulging buttocks

Personally, I used to eat these 'complex carbs' all the time, mostly because we were told to base our diet on such foods.

- Cereals and toast for breakfast
- Sandwiches or filled rolls/baguette for lunch
- Pasta or rice or spaghetti for dinner

These are the energy foods, we were told to fill up on these low-calorie, bulky, slow-burn carbs that give us 'slow release' energy all day. The government dietary advice for weight loss in the 80s and 90s and still today was to bulk out your diet with lots of these foods, so you get an even supply of energy all day long. WRONG!

Personally, of my 101 pounds of weight loss, a good 20 or 30 pounds of it came from just quitting these carbs. No other lifestyle change, I just quit bread and pasta, and lost 20 or 30 pounds in about five months.

All the time, I meet friends who say to me something like: "Karl, I just haven't got time to come to your seminar, or listen to you shout enthusiastically for an hour-and-a-half about broccoli, so just give your top tip in 60 seconds, how can I lose some weight?"

And I always reply with something along the lines of: "Just give up cereals, bread and pasta. Let me know how it goes in six months." And the vast majority of those people call me or email a few months later saying, 'I've just lost 20 pounds! All I did was cut out bread.'

Try it. Cut out the breakfast cereals, the toast, the sandwiches, all those cakes and pastries, the pizza bases, that 'comfort meal' bowl of pasta with cheese grated on it, the heaps of white rice and white potatoes; that stuff is all making you fat. Unless you are an athlete, you just don't need all those carbs.

Maybe for a handful of very active people, avid marathon runners, bodybuilders, outside labourers, these physical hard workers, maybe they need more carbs, but they are a small minority of people. Most people I meet who need to lose some weight work inside all day and most sit down all day. We are told to eat starchy carbohydrates for energy – well how much energy do you need to sit on your butt all day long?

Slow release' energy from complex carbs. Seriously, how much energy do you need to sit on your butt all day?

Because so many people now eat these foods as 'the bulk' element of a meal (think cereals and toast for breakfast, sandwiches for lunch, pasta, rice and spaghetti for dinner – see, the starchy carbs are providing the bulk of the meal time and again) this can often lead to over-eating large quantities of these foods.

Because of this issue of quantity, these grains and starchy carbs tend to contribute a substantial proportion of the calories in a person's diet, but comparatively little micronutrients (vitamins and minerals). This is all contributing to weight gain and a situation where folks are 'over-fed but under-nourished', which is fast becoming the curse of our society.

Insulin sensitivity

All carbs, including 'complex carbs' are broken down inside your body to simple sugars that your body can digest and use. Eating lots of these sugars leads to a release of insulin in your body, which serves many useful functions, but it also causes the excess sugars from all these starchy carbs to be stored as body fat, unless there is an immediate physical need for that energy. (Nutrition graduates please forgive my scientific brevity!)

Over and over, day after day, this repeated cycle of eating carbs, and releasing insulin, and storing excess energy as body fay, all leads to unwanted weight gain, obesity, and eventually a blunting of this insulin response. This can contribute to insulin resistance and metabolic syndrome, and a growing body of evidence suggests this is exacerbating rates of type-2 diabetes.

Being overweight or obese is the **second largest preventable cause of cancer in the UK**, according to Cancer Research UK. A very substantial five percent of cancer in the UK is caused by people being overweight and obese. In our age of political correctness, we are all scared of talking about 'being fat' these days for fear we might offend someone. I understand the good reasons to end 'fat shaming' and stop bullying and negative stereotypes around body image, but I worry this is all moving us to make obesity more of a socially acceptable norm.

If you are overweight or obese, you are still a beautiful and lovable person and a valuable member of society, no one should have their character judged for being overweight, **but your health is suffering from your excess bodyweight**, and we must be careful not to confuse issues of *health*, with issues of beauty, bullying and social acceptance.

However, let's not just blame starchy carbs and sugar for making people overweight, and don't blame insulin either! Insulin is just a hormone, one we can't live without, and it's just doing its job. If someone is overweight, they have been taking in more calories than they have been using – starchy carbs and refined sugar are just 'component parts' of the problem!

Gluten

There are compounds in grains – gluten, lectins, phytic acid and enzyme inhibitors – that are undesirable and have negative side-effects inside your body. These compounds can contribute to all manner of digestive disorders and autoimmune problems. A lot of people suffer from gluten sensitivity but they are not aware of it.

I am purposefully keeping this brief here, but if you suffer any digestive issues, bloating, gas, or inflammatory conditions (that could mean anything from skin conditions, to heart disease, from nasal congestion to arthritis) then it could possibly be that gluten is the cause, or a factor in aggravating the condition. If you suffer from any digestive health problems or inflammatory conditions, you may benefit from trying six months off grains to see if it makes a positive difference to your life.

For a great number of people, the most common sign of an issue is farting! If you eat a meal and it leaves you feeling bloated, gassy, feeling like you just want to be alone somewhere so you can fart for all you're worth, that's a classic sign you are eating gluten and your gut would rather you didn't.

Micronutrients – vitamins and minerals

If you are eating lots of starchy carbs, chances are you're not packing in other more nutritious foods that your body could use to help you achieve supreme good health – such as lots of vegetables. It's not to say "rice is bad for you" or "there are no vitamins in bread" but it's broadly true that these starchy carbs are comparatively low in micronutrients when compared to more nutritious foods such as vegetables, fish and so on.

> # These starchy carbs are displacing more nutritious foods from your diet.

In the next chapter, you will learn more about the importance of vitamins and minerals, and how they help us to have more energy, look and feel our best, resist ill health and resist the signs of ageing. Personally, I'll have a serving of mackerel and six or seven servings of green veg for my breakfast. I've got more nutrients in my diet by 9am than most people eat all day. But that's me! Let's just take this one step at a time…

Food swaps

Someone's going to look at this and think, "Oh no, he's going to take my bread away." Yep. Sorry. It's for your own good! The question I am most often asked is this, "But if I have to give up cereals and toast, what the heck am I supposed to eat for breakfast?"

OK, I did say a couple of chapters back that you would have to face making some changes, that things might get a little uncomfortable. Remember, **if you keep doing what you've been doing, you'll keep getting what you've been getting**. I'm not going to pretend that I put the *Crunchy Nut Cornflakes* down one day, and had mackerel and cabbage the next. It didn't happen that fast, I didn't have the 12 Core Principles of *Mother Nature's Diet* to guide me through this change in my life a decade ago; I had to figure it out for myself. My transition happened slowly over a number of years.

I went from cereal and toast to fresh fruit, then to a breakfast smoothie, which in time became scrambled eggs, which then became scrambled eggs with a couple of handfuls of spinach thrown in. The scrambled eggs with spinach, became scrambled eggs with broccoli in, and then with cabbage in, then the eggs came out, and the cabbage stayed, and the mackerel came along. And what do you know, we've made it to cabbage and mackerel for breakfast, in seven progressive steps, which probably took three or four years. One step at a time.

Let's look at some simple food swaps you can make to get the bulk of these processed carbs out of your diet…without leaping straight to mackerel and cabbage in one hit!

Breakfast

OUT: Cereals, toast, bagels, baps, waffles and pancakes.
IN: Scrambled eggs; bacon and eggs; fresh fruit or a smoothie.
With some practice, I have got the art of knocking up scrambled eggs with a couple of handfuls of spinach in it down to about four minutes. If you haven't

got four minutes to make breakfast, you need to re-evaluate your life priorities. I'm serious, your good health matters.

Lunch

OUT: bread - sandwiches and filled rolls, wraps or baguettes.
IN: salad, lots of lovely colourful salad.
This is an easy swap to make. Anything you would normally put in a sandwich, put it on a salad instead.

> ➤ If you would normally mash up tuna with mayonnaise and spread that in a sandwich
>> ➤ Just mash up the tuna and put it on a salad instead
> ➤ Slices of ham or chicken?
>> ➤ Cut them up on a salad instead
> ➤ Hard boiled eggs, mashed in a sandwich?
>> ➤ Slice them on a salad instead
> ➤ Cheese in a sandwich?
>> ➤ Chunks of cheese on a salad instead

See how easy this is? After a few days practice, you'll be able to knock up a box of salad as quickly as you can make a sandwich. Some people tell me they don't make their own lunch, they buy it in the local shop. Well in my experience most of the places where they sell filled sandwiches and filled baguettes, they also sell boxed salads. Where there's a will, there's a way. Yes?

Dinner

OUT: pasta, rice, spaghetti, masses of white potatoes.
IN: vegetables! Lots of lovely veggies!
Anywhere you would normally use rice, pasta or spaghetti, you can use more vegetables instead. It's easy. Maybe it's a bit weird. Your partner, spouse, loved one, housemates and colleagues might think you're a bit of a freak for about the first week, but they'll soon get used to it.

I still make spaghetti Bolognese, only I make **broccoli Bolognese**. I just make the Bolognese, and then instead of boiling a pan of spaghetti, I steam a pan full of broccoli. I just put the broccoli on the plate, and the Bolognese beside it. It's an easy swap. You see how simple this is? Instead of boiling one thing (spaghetti) for ten minutes, I steam something else (broccoli) in its place for ten minutes. Done, everything else is the same. You see, no one can say that's hard, the meal takes no longer to prepare, it's no more complicated, just one simple ingredient swapped for another.

I will still make a **chilli-con-carne**, but instead of putting it on a bed of white rice, I'll put it on a bed of cabbage, broccoli, or cauliflower. Again, that's a dead simple swap, instead of boiling a pan of rice, boil a pan of cauliflower. No extra effort at all. If you want to get all fancy, then Google how to make 'cauliflower rice' and you can even fool your family into thinking it looks like white rice!

Another option is **'courgetti spaghetti'**. You can buy a gadget called a spiralizer, which allows you to make courgettes look like spaghetti. You can then prepare courgetti spaghetti even faster than boiling the spaghetti itself...the courgette only requires about one minute in boiling water to be ready. Or you can flash fry it in just a few minutes with a knob of butter and some paprika, it's very tasty. You can also spiralize carrots, and other vegetables. There are several restaurant chains across the UK now offering courgetti spaghetti on the menu, on all their pasta dishes, which is great progress.

I still make a curry, but instead of putting it on basmati rice, I'll put it on **cauliflower**, or broccoli. You see, it's actually pretty easy to make these swaps. Wherever you would normally have a big heap of pasta, spaghetti, rice or white potatoes, just switch all that starch out for lots of nutritious veggies instead.

Best of the rest

When I talk about cutting these carbs in my live seminars, someone will almost always come up to me in the break and ask me about oats. There are certain grains and starches that are 'best of a bad lot' for want of a better expression. For clarity, it's worth understanding that:

- If cheap sliced white bread is the worst end of 'the bread spectrum', then organic, fermented sourdough bread is the far other end of that spectrum, the healthy end
- If the worst end of the breakfast cereal spectrum is Choco-covered-wheat-crispy-shite, then plain organic oats is the far opposite end, the good end, less sugar and more micronutrients

- If a filled white soft roll is the worst end of the lunch spectrum, then I guess an organic gluten-free whole wheat wrap is the best possible option, if no salad is available
- If a huge bowl of white pasta is the bad end of the starchy carbs spectrum at dinner, then a modest serving of quinoa is pretty much at the other end of that scale

Can you see? It's all on a scale. **There's bread, and then there's bread.** One is nutritionally hollow, lacking much goodness and packed with added sugar, the other can be a healthy part of a balanced diet. But seriously, how many people do you know who regularly eat organic, fermented sourdough bread? Compared to how many people buy a sliced loaf in the supermarket? You see? The easiest broad advice to give is "ditch the bread".

So, can I eat sourdough bread and quinoa?

If you are trying to lose a bunch of weight, and if your work/life is largely sedentary, then I still suggest you cut those carbs...at least until you hit your bodyweight goals and stabilise at a weight and lifestyle balance you are happy with. If you're not trying to lose weight, you never suffer gastrointestinal discomfort, bloating, or gas after eating starchy foods, and you're in good shape, and you don't have any autoimmune problems, and you just enjoy oats a couple of times a week because it helps you fuel a run or a gym session, then I'd say, oats are okay, go for it.

Most of the time, you can get your carbs from more nutritious foods, like sweet potato, butternut squash, nuts, bananas, pumpkin, cauliflower, and other fruits and veggies.

Summary

There are many good reasons not to eat grains...and there are many better food choices available! If we look at the major health challenges our society faces today, we can see that rising obesity rates and rising type-2 diabetes rates are both close to the top of the list. Meanwhile, too many people are eating too much processed food, high in sugar and low in micronutrients.

What we need is less bulky 'beige food' that is high in calories but low in nutrients. We need to eat less of that stuff, and more fresh, whole foods, high in nutrients.

> It's a shift to fewer calories, more nutrients.
> It's less food, more nourishment, and that's what many people need.

What have we learned in this chapter?

- For most people, eating too much bread, cereals and pasta is making them fat. As well as contributing to rising obesity, these starchy carbs are contributing to the rise in type-2 diabetes too
- Eliminating grains and starchy processed carbs from your diet and eating lots more fresh vegetables instead, is a sensible substitution, aimed at improving the nutrient density of your diet – see the next chapter for more on this
- MND Core Principle 1 recommends "Quit the grains and starchy carbs" as broad advice to the public as a whole – and that is very different from saying "never eat these foods, they are really bad for you"
- There are a bunch of exceptions to this 'Rule' – if you're a bodybuilder or weight lifter, you probably eat lots of carbs, and you probably know what you're doing, so that's cool, good for you. Maybe you run marathons and you love eating tons of carbs, and you burn it all off every week, well good for you, if you are gluten tolerant and that works for you then you could keep doing that if you want to
- But bodybuilders and marathon runners only make up, maybe, 2% of our population. For most other folks, cutting back on these starchy carbs is probably a good idea, especially if you want to lose some weight. Whatever activity you do, you will likely benefit from making some better choices

- Breakfast cereals, bread and pasta are low-nutrient carbohydrate options, and you could be getting your carbs from sweet potato, squash and parsnips, foods which will give you additional micronutrients, and foods that don't come with added sugar, processed salt and other additives
- Anecdotally, many people trying to lose weight report that the single best thing they have done to quickly shift persistent undesirable body fat is to drop grains and starchy carbs. Unless you're an athlete, quit bread and pasta for three to six months and see the weight come off for you too

Sidebar: Micronutrients

I n the previous chapter we looked at swapping these bulky, starchy carbs that make up such a hefty proportion of many people's diet, for more nutritious foods, such as fresh vegetables and oily fish. I promised to explain the importance of vitamins and minerals in our diet. That's what we are going to look at in this chapter.

Vitamins and minerals

I am sure you have heard of vitamins and minerals, and it's probably safe to say that you know *something* about them - what they are, what they do. So, think about it, what do you **really know** about vitamins and minerals? I don't know about you, but until I started learning about nutrition in my mid-30s, this roughly sums up what I knew as a young adult:

- Vitamins and minerals are compounds found in certain foods
- They're good for you!
- They help you to have good skin, hair, teeth and nails
- Beta-carotene (makes carrots orange in colour) helps you see in the dark. I think, maybe, that I knew that beta-carotene had something to do with vitamin A
- Calcium is good for your teeth and bones
- Iron makes your blood 'strong and healthy' – people with low iron get anaemia
- Vitamin C helps fight off coughs and colds. Low vitamin C causes scurvy, which used to kill sailors many years ago
- Some vitamins are called antioxidants, these are supposed to help you be healthy and fight off ill health in lots of ways

That's about it. In the first 35 years of my life, that pretty much sums up what I learned about vitamins and minerals. I'm guessing this information came mostly from my mum, or maybe they told us these things at school, and maybe I picked up a couple of bottles on the shelf in the health food shop and read the labels.

What about you? Are you looking at my list and thinking "Is that all you knew, I know loads more than that!" or are you thinking "Yup, I'm about the same as you pal?" Or maybe you're thinking "Oh I didn't know that! Some of this is new to me."

What else do we know? When I cover this topic in live seminars, I ask my audience what they know, I ask them to shout out. They usually cover the same things as I have in that list, above, and then sometimes they get a few extras such as:

- Vitamin A is good for your eyesight
- Vitamin C for your immune system (I had that one on my list!)
- Vitamin D for teeth and bones (it helps us to absorb and use calcium)
- Vitamin E for good skin

Generally, that's about it. Sometimes I have biologists or medically trained people in my audience, doctors, dentists, nurses, surgeons, and so sometimes (but very rarely indeed) I also get these:

- B Group vitamins help with energy production
- Some vitamins and minerals help our body to digest and assimilate other vitamins and minerals
- For example, vitamin C helps us to absorb iron
- Vitamin K helps with calcium and absorption
- A vitamin D deficiency can cause Rickets

And that just about sums up what most people, the British public, know about vitamins and minerals. But actually, there's a bit more to it than that.

What my mum didn't tell me, likely because she didn't know, just like all the people in every room I have spoken to in live seminars over the last five years didn't know either, was that all the 13 vitamins and 15 minerals that we need from our diet, are essential, they are *vital*. I mean, without them, **without any one of them**, you would die. And to be honest, that's seriously going to spoil your day.

Death, and other slightly-less-serious health concerns

Wow, so it turns out these little vitamins and minerals are a whole bunch more important than my mum let on. I guess she didn't know, we'll give her the benefit of the doubt on that one.

Let's dig a little deeper. Most folks know that a vitamin C deficiency can lead to scurvy. The first symptom of scurvy is bleeding gums. It's often the dentist who first notices that there is a problem. But here's the interesting thing. Scurvy is in fact a disease of 'leaking blood vessels' and so it shows up in your gums quite early on because that's the first place visible from the outside of a human body where 'leaking arteries' can be seen, because the skin/tissues between the arteries in your gums, and the exterior world is thinnest there.

However, inside your body, other blood vessels will soon start leaking too, until you die of internal bleeding. In order to maintain healthy collagen synthesis (collagen is an important structural protein, and your blood vessels and skin are largely made of collagen) you need plenty of vitamin C. If you run short, your blood vessels start springing leaks, and you bleed to death internally. (Apologies to doctors and biologists for the simplicity!)

It seems to me then, that aiding collagen synthesis, is an extremely important function of vitamin C. But beyond that, good old vitamin C also does some other, shall we say 'less important' things, such as supporting immune function, and helping keep blood pressure stable.

Now, it seems to me that we could probably draw some kind of graph or chart or graphic here, showing how vitamin C is good for you.

- At the bottom we might show 'no' vitamin C = death
- Up a little way we could show 'very little' vitamin C = very sick with scurvy
- Up a little way from that we could show 'little' vitamin C = feeling weary and bleeding gums
- Up a little further might show 'low' levels of vitamin C = not bad enough for scurvy, but feeling weary, tired all the time, poor immune system function
- Up further still we might show 'average' level of vitamin C = no obvious illness, feel OK, feel average

Let's illustrate this as a little graphic and see how it looks…

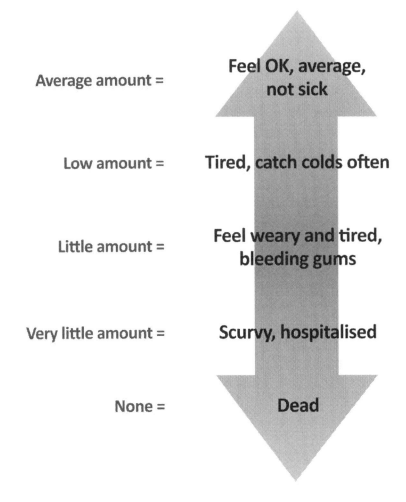

Average amount = **Feel OK, average, not sick**

Low amount = **Tired, catch colds often**

Little amount = **Feel weary and tired, bleeding gums**

Very little amount = **Scurvy, hospitalised**

None = **Dead**

OK, so clearly, I'm not going to win any major industry awards for my graphic design skills, but can you see this concept, can you see how this works?

Now at this point, I hope you are starting to change how you think about vitamins and minerals. We all knew that we needed 'some' vitamin C to be healthy. We all knew that if we ate a shockingly poor diet and became terribly vitamin C deficient then we would develop scurvy, and our gums would bleed. But did you know that untreated, you would then die from that scurvy? And did you realise that **there might be this kind of 'sliding scale' of health**, depending on how much vitamin C you were getting?

Get an average amount, and feel average, but as your vitamin C levels decline, so does your health, all the way down to death. Are you learning something here?

Now, what if I told you – we could pretty much draw the same graphic for all 13 essential vitamins, and all 15 essential minerals – how would that change what you think of these little micronutrients then?

Vitamin A – average amount, you can see OK. Get a bit low, start to lose night vision. Get lower, go blind. Down to zero, you die. Sadly, vitamin A deficiency (VAD) is the leading preventable cause of blindness in children worldwide, and in the developing world, over 300,000 children go blind every year from VAD, and around half of them die.[1]

Vitamin B1 – aids with energy production, metabolism, nervous system function and many other important jobs. If you get an average amount of it, you'll feel fine, average. If you run low, you will suffer fatigue and more, if you run really low you'll develop a disease called beriberi, and if you 'zero out' completely, you'll die.[2]

Vitamin B3 – same as B1 and others in B Group, aids energy production, metabolism and nervous system function. If you run low you develop pellagra, and untreated, you'll die.[3]

Iron – essential for building proteins, aids energy production, builds red blood cells and helps immune system. Get an average amount, you'll feel average. Run low, you'll feel tired and weak and develop anaemia. Zero out completely, and you'll die.

Vitamin D - same story...
Calcium - same again...
Sodium - same...
Zinc - same...

---

[1] Vitamin A deficiency. https://en.wikipedia.org/wiki/Vitamin_A_deficiency
[2] Thiamine deficiency. https://en.wikipedia.org/wiki/Thiamine_deficiency
[3] Pellagra. https://en.wikipedia.org/wiki/Pellagra

I could do this all day long. The point is this. All 28 vitamins and minerals are the same, they all fit that graphic on the previous page, they all tell the same story of the sliding scale.

- 13 vitamins
- 15 minerals
- If you have an average amount, you'll feel average, OK
- **If you go 'a bit low' you'll start to feel a bit crappy**
- If you go 'very low' you'll be horribly sick
- If you bottom out to 'none' you will die

[Note: Please, PhDs in biochemistry, dietitians and nutritional therapists, I know this is a drastic over-simplification, but cut me some slack here, I am trying to keep this interesting, relevant and easy-going! Thanks!]

Obviously, there is some broad variation, but in general terms, all 28 of these essential micronutrients fit this same model, they all fit on this sliding scale.

Now all these vitamins and minerals do a multitude of useful jobs inside us. Many of them have what we might think of as 'primary functions' and then many of them also have 'lesser functions'. For example, vitamin C helps with collagen synthesis, so that keeps our blood vessels intact, a pretty primary function of vitamin C I would say. In fact, collagen is the most ubiquitous protein in the human body (and there are many hundreds of thousands of proteins in a human body) and it is a major component of human skin.

Vitamin C, therefore, is also good for your skin, and another one of the early signs of scurvy, is poor skin, with little red or purple spots, skin haemorrhages and lesions, and poor wound healing. Further symptoms of a vitamin C deficiency might include fatigue, tiredness, weakness, irritability and poor immune function (catching lots of coughs and colds all the time.)

Can you imagine now, how we could fit all those symptoms onto our sliding scale? Let's draw another little graphic to see what that might look like.

Average amount =	**Feel OK, average, not sick**
	Lethargic
	Weary, irritable
Low amount =	**Tired, catch colds often**
	Poor skin, flu, bugs
	Bad skin, constant colds
Little amount =	**Feel weary and tired, bleeding gums**
	Skin lesions
	Anaemia and weakness
Very little amount =	**Scurvy, hospitalised**
	Need treatment...
	Otherwise...
None =	**Dead**

Can you see how perhaps a mild deficiency can cause mild illness – weary, irritable, get lots of coughs and colds, tired all the time, crappy skin, look and feel a bit rubbish for your age. **Can you see that?** (Or have you gone off to get a grapefruit or an orange to top up your vitamin C? Or are you busy checking your skin for red spots and blotches?)

It's the same with vitamin A. Sure, helping you to have good eyesight and helping to prevent blindness is a primary function of vitamin A, but it has many secondary functions too, including helping to boost your immune system, helping you to have good skin, and helping you to make good healthy red blood cells.

If we made a 'sliding scale graphic' for vitamin A like the one for vitamin C, while we would see "OK and average" at the top and we'd see "dead" at the bottom, and "blind" above it, what we might see in the "a little bit low" area might include poor immune function, failing eyesight and crappy skin.

Now, for both the vitamin C and vitamin A example, can you see how these symptoms of being "a little bit low" on these nutrients are actually really quite common complaints that in fact a fair majority of the population frequently complain about?

- Lethargy
- Weariness
- Tired all the time
- Not much energy
- Sick and tired of feeling sick and tired
- Ageing poorly – bad skin, bad hair, bad nails, eyesight failing
- Brain fog, irritability, concentration problems
- Poor immune function, catch colds all the time

These are common conditions, common complaints. I can tell you, I suffered from those complaints when I was 'old me' – the fat unhealthy guy with a poor diet. I don't suffer from any of those things now! **Ummm...that's something to ponder, isn't it?**

One of the things that gives us plenty of energy is *healthy ATP production* (don't worry about what ATP is, it's a molecule, it's a 'unit of energy' to your muscles) and another thing is good *healthy red blood cells*, these carry oxygen around the body which supplies oxygen to working muscles and organs. So, if you have good healthy red blood cells, and good healthy ATP production, you should have plenty of energy.

We've already seen that both vitamin A and iron play an important role in *red blood cell production*, as do vitamins B9 and B12. And we know that most of the B Group vitamins *play a role in ATP production*, that's energy production. If we drew our little 'sliding scale' graphics for vitamin A, iron, B1, B2, B3, B5, B9 and B12 – we would see how being 'a bit low' on any or all of these, could result in feeling weary, tired, lethargic, **lacking in energy** or vitality.

According to a number of surveys carried out between 2008 and 2015, lacking energy and feeling tired all the time is the single most common health complaint among UK adults in the 21st century! **Ummm...something further to ponder!!**

Maybe everyone's just eating a crappy diet?!?!?!

Let's see. Let's explore that thought, just briefly. Have you heard of the RDA of a vitamin or mineral? It means 'Recommended Daily Allowance' or 'Recommended Daily Amount' or 'Recommended Dietary Amount'. In some countries it is called RDI, 'Recommended Dietary Intake' or 'Reference Daily Intake'. Lots of ways of saying roughly the same thing.

Do you know what this is and what it means? These are the values of vitamins and minerals in food products, and the amount our government suggest you should eat every day or week. When you look at the nutrition label on packaged food, it tells you that eating a certain amount of that food (one serving, or 100 grams) you will get xx% of your RDA of certain vitamins and minerals. Have you seen this?

Here's a definition for you:

> **Recommended Dietary Allowance:** The RDA, the estimated amount of a nutrient per day considered necessary for the maintenance of good health by the Food and Nutrition Board of the National Research Council/ National Academy of Sciences.
> http://www.nationalacademies.org/nasem/

The government establish RDAs for these micronutrients, minimum amounts we should consume to "maintain good health" whatever that means. I did some looking in to what that does actually mean. How do you think they established these needs?

Do you think they sat down with all the Olympic silver and gold winners for the last 20 years and said, "Let's look at the dietary requirements of gold medal winning Olympians and recommend that diet for everyone."? Do you think that's how they did it?

Do you think they gathered all the people in the UK in the 1970s who lived to 95 and above, or all the people who made it to 100 without developing heart disease or cancer, and tested them and measured their diet as the 'target base line' for us all to live? Do you think that's the standard they worked to?

Or do you think they went to the hospitals and they got all the sick people dying of scurvy, pellagra and beriberi, and studied their diet, and set these RDA targets from there?

No, of course not, they didn't do any of those things. They calculate RDAs based on research studies, lab studies on human nutrition, and they calculate the "average needs of the average person" required "to maintain good health" meaning "to not get sick", and then these become our RDA guidelines. They do not base these guidelines on Olympians, elite athletes, people who live to over 100 years of age, or any specially selected samples of the fittest, healthiest, strongest people. They base these figures on the needs of the average person.

So, let me ask you a question - look around you, look at our society, and tell me...

"Is your goal in life to be average?"

I don't know about you, and I am not being judgemental here, but I look around me and I see the *average* person struggling with their weight, struggling with tiredness, struggling for energy, struggling with ageing, I see the *average* person getting multiple coughs and colds every year, complaining of feeling weary and afraid of chronic degenerative disease in old age, and I mean heart disease and cancer.

I look around me, and I want to be doing a lot better than **average**.

How about you?

Government guidelines

I think it's important to remember that the government's 'job' (for want of a better descriptive word) is to try to prevent people from suffering ill health, sickness and premature death. The government has an interest in trying to ensure that we, the people, are not all dying young of some nasty disease, but that doesn't mean it's the government's job to "make you feel freakin' awesome" or "to ensure you age gracefully and have beautiful soft skin" or "to ensure you are slim, vibrant, energetic, attractive, happy and full of beans".

Right? I mean come on, we have this amazing NHS that is free at the point of entry, it's there to fix us up after a car crash; help us deliver babies; your doctor is there for you every week if you need him or her; the NHS is there for all our emergencies and surgeries and truly they are absolute heroes and they do an amazing job. World class in my opinion. But it's really not their job to come around and knock on your door every couple of years and help you firm up your buttocks, lose a couple of inches off your waist, get a new haircut and look fabulous.

No! If you want to look fabulous, shape up and feel fantastic, tone up your mid-section and look and feel great for your age, that's your job!

It's your responsibility. It's down to you.

In short: the NHS, and the Department of Health and Social Care, are there to treat sickness and injury, and 99% of their budget, time and resources go on just that. There is actually very little resource allocated to promoting good health, to stopping folks getting sick in the first place.

Of course, there are lots of health and safety laws to try to prevent accidents. We have to wear seat belts in cars, there are speed limits on our roads, and cars have air bags fitted. There are rules and regulations around electrical wiring, fuse boxes, safety barriers, fences, hand rails and so on. These measures are there to prevent accidents and injuries.

What about advice for staying healthy? There are a variety of recommendations that we see promoted quite widely.

- Eat your **5-a-day**
- Drink aware. Enjoy alcohol responsibly. **Safe limits**
- **Don't smoke** / stop smoking
- **Eat fish**, especially oily fish, twice per week[4]
- The Eatwell Plate or **The Eatwell Guide** and our **RDAs** of vitamins and minerals[5]

---

[4] NHS website: https://www.nhs.uk/live-well/eat-well/fish-and-shellfish-nutrition/
[5] The Eatwell Guide: https://www.gov.uk/government/publications/the-eatwell-guide

The Eatwell *Guide* is the newly-updated guide that came out in 2016. Prior to that, from 1994 until 2016, the UK was told to follow The Eatwell *Plate* – a picture that was promoted widely and taught to our children in school. If anything represents 'the official government guidelines' during the years when this obesity epidemic and type-2 diabetes epidemic became reality, it's The Eatwell Plate. While The Eatwell *Guide* is what they share now, The Eatwell *Plate* is very much 'what got us to here' so far.

The eatwell plate

Use the eatwell plate to help you get the balance right. It shows how much of what you eat should come from each food group.

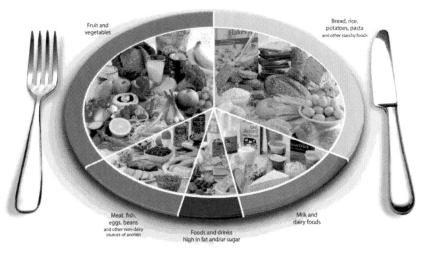

Public Health England in association with the Welsh Government, the Scottish Government and the Food Standards Agency in Northern Ireland

The picture shows The Eatwell Plate, which includes: Corn flakes, Weetabix (or a similar brand), white rice, white bread rolls, white bagel, white pasta, white spaghetti, white potatoes, white pita breads, soft white rolls, sliced white bread, white and brown sliced bread mixed together.

We've also got soya milk, little fruit-flavoured, low-fat yoghurt pots (several teaspoons of sugar in every pot), we see fizzy cola, crisps, Victoria sponge cake, Battenberg cake, custard cream biscuits, chocolate Bourbon biscuits, cheap vegetable/seed oil, chocolate chip cookies, jelly sweets, something that looks like Smarties or M&M's and a bar of chocolate. All those things making up almost half of what you see, and then what I call real food – meat, fish, vegetables, fruits, eggs and nuts making up the other half.

This image has been our national healthy eating guide through the 90's and into the 21st century, for some 22 years.

What are people actually doing?

Are folks actually following all this advice? Do the British public eat their 5-a-day? **Nope.** The reality is, only 27% of adults in the UK actually eat their five-a-day. Whenever I ask a live audience, by show of hands, about one third of the room claim to eat their 5-a-day. Two-thirds of the nation, 73% of the population, are not getting their five-a-day.[6]

Many scientists warn that five-a-day is too low. Our own government have been lobbied repeatedly by scientists saying we should raise it to at least **seven-a-day**. It's proven to have better cancer fighting benefits.[7] Many argue we should aim for 10-a-day, or even more.[8] There's a lot of other countries out there promoting seven-a-day or more, so here in the UK we're really not setting the bar very high at 5-a-day. And sadly, still almost three-quarters of the population aren't hitting that low bar.

Remember, what is that advice we are given, for us to avoid disease and stay healthy?

- Eat your **5-a-day**
- Drinkaware. Enjoy alcohol responsibly. **Safe limits**
- **Don't smoke** / stop smoking
- **Eat fish**, especially oily fish, twice per week
- The Eat Well Plate or **The Eatwell Guide** and our **RDA**s of vitamins and minerals

Let's take a look at these one by one.

---

[6] *Adults who eat five or more portions of fruit and vegetables per day.* Trends 2001-2017. http://healthsurvey.hscic.gov.uk/data-visualisation/data-visualisation/explore-the-trends/fruit-vegetables.aspx
[7] Oyebode, O., et al. (2014). Fruit and vegetable consumption and all-cause, cancer and CVD mortality: analysis of Health Survey for England data. *Journal of Epidemiology & Community Health* 2014; 68 799-800. Published Online First: 31 Mar 2014. Retrieved from https://jech.bmj.com/content/68/9/856.short
[8] https://www.telegraph.co.uk/news/2017/02/23/five-a-day-fruit-veg-must-double-10-major-study-finds/

5-a-day: Right, so a lot of scientists argue that 5-a-day is too low, and yet most (73% of people) are not even eating that. Clearly, there's room for improvement there.

Alcohol: The Drinkaware campaign, and the high cost of drinking alcohol in pubs, clubs and restaurants, has made some progress, but overall binge drinking culture has risen in the UK in the past 30 years. In late 2015 the government lowered safe drinking limits[9], though still around a quarter of British adults drink too many units per week.[10]

Smoking: Stop smoking – this has been a great success, since the 1960s when over 80% of British men smoked, now it's down to under 20%. The NHS offers a proven smoking cessation program that helps lots of people to quit. Bravo!

Fish: Does the average Brit east fish twice a week? Well, not in the audiences I ask, and according to a 2011 survey, only 28% of the British public eat fish twice per week.

Diet: And the Eatwell Plate, as we discussed above, recommends half your diet comes from starchy processed carbs and sugary snacks! See MND Core Principle 1 and Core Principle 2 for everything that's wrong with that, and for how that may have contributed massively to the rise in obesity and type-2 diabetes over the last 20 years!

In summary, where are the British public, in terms of following this advice from the Department of Health and Social care? Well, two thirds don't eat enough fruits and veggies; two thirds don't eat enough fish; 20% still smoke; about a third or so still drink too much; and those who do follow the recommended diet, in my opinion, are probably eating too many processed carbs and too much sugar.

Add to that the fact that only 30% of British women and 40% of British men get the recommended minimum amount of exercise, and that's another low-set bar in my opinion (See Core Principle 9, later in this book)

---

[9] Drinkaware, see https://www.drinkaware.co.uk/alcohol-facts/alcoholic-drinks-units/latest-uk-alcohol-unit-guidance/
[10] The Guardian: *Weekly alcohol limit cut to 14 units in UK for men.* https://www.theguardian.com/society/2016/jan/08/mens-recommended-maximum-weekly-alcohol-units-cut-14

and the fact that 75% of the British public are vitamin D deficient because folks all work inside these days and don't get enough sunlight (see Core Principle 11, later in this book) and overall, it's not a good situation. Actually, it's all pretty worrying, and hardly surprising that so many people are not in optimum good health.

> It's not unrealistic to say that a staggering three quarters of the British population eat a poor diet, high in processed, low-nutrient foods and sugar, but low in oily fish, fresh vegetables and fruits, and they are likely slightly deficient in a number of vitamins and minerals.
>
> Frankly, that sucks.

People often say to me that they really don't think that diet is that much of a big deal. They don't think the whole 5-a-day thing is particularly important, they think you can eat pretty much anything they sell in supermarkets and you'll be fine. (Remember, most folks think vitamins 'give you nice hair and skin' and that's about all they know.)

According to Cancer Research UK, in 2017, poor diet is the third largest preventable cause of cancer in the UK, contributing to between 5% and 10% of UK cancers. CRUK stated in 2015, that 9% of cancers in the UK could be prevented just by people eating their 5-a-day, **or more**, and reducing the amount of processed foods in their diet.

Still think diet is no big deal now?

Triage theory

There is a brilliant scientist called Dr Bruce Ames who postulated 'the triage theory of nutrient allocation' back in 2006.[11] Cutting some pretty complex

---

[11] Ames, B.N. (2006). Low micronutrient intake may accelerate the degenerative diseases of aging through allocation of scarce micronutrients by triage. *PNAS* November 21, 2006 103 (47) 17589-17594. https://doi.org/10.1073/pnas.0608757103

'science rather short, the excellent Dr Ames suggested that our bodies allocate scarce resources, such as an inadequate supply of micronutrients, on a sort-of 'triage' basis. That is to say…

> *If there's not enough of something to go around, we'll allocate what there is to the most urgent and important jobs first, and then see what's left. If we then don't have enough for all the less important jobs, oh well, try again tomorrow!*

Now think again, if your body didn't have enough vitamin C to do all its jobs, wouldn't you think it might prioritise the important stuff, like not letting your arteries burst and leak and you bleed to death…it might allocate what vitamin C is available to collagen synthesis, and screw the rest. Yep, that's exactly what it does.

So, you eat a poor diet all week…you don't get scurvy, well yippee, but you didn't have enough vitamin C left to work on the immune system, so you feel a bit crap, you don't have much energy, and you catch a cold. Can you see where that fits on our **sliding scale graphic**? Not bad enough to wind up in hospital, just not good enough to really thrive and feel great.

Pulling it all together

I am sorry, things have become fragmented and it may seem as if we have jumped around all over the place. Let's tie all these strands together, everything we have looked at in this chapter.

- Vitamins and minerals are good for you. Very good for you. Without any, you die. With a low supply, you get sick. If your intake is 'just a bit low' you might look and feel like crap, you may be ageing badly, you might be low on energy and be prone to ill health
- RDAs are set to help you achieve 'average' health and not get sick, they are hardly 'aspirational goals for feeling awesome'
- I'm not sure we all aspire to 'averageness' as a major life goal…?
- The government recommend we eat 5-a-day – three quarters of people don't
- They recommend we drink moderately at most – half the nation drink a bit too much (alcohol depletes some of these minerals in your gut, so even if you are eating them in your diet, you then may not be

absorbing them all, not if that nutritious dinner is washed down with two glasses of wine like mine always used to be)

- The government recommend that we eat highly nutritious fish at least twice per week, but three quarters of people don't
- Around 65% of people also don't get enough exercise, and around 75% of people don't get enough sunlight and are somewhat vitamin D deficient (vitamin D comes from sun exposure and oily fish in your diet)
- The triage theory says that if we are somewhat deficient in a vitamin or mineral, then our body will use what is available for the most life-threateningly essential jobs, and then leave the less important jobs (like good skin, eyes, hair, energy production, fighting coughs and colds)
- Putting all this together, it's easy to see how three quarters of the British population are basically eating a crappy diet, and they are likely falling short of hitting these RDA targets for achieving 'average health'
- The result of these minor (I call them sub-clinical, meaning you don't end up in hospital for it) nutrient deficiencies is low energy, poor immune function, coughs and colds, bugs and chest infections, poor ageing, bad skin, hair, weak nails, deteriorating eyesight, brain fog, irritability, and so on
- Maybe, as we age, this poor metabolic function and poor immune function is also contributing to chronic degenerative disease, such as diabetes, heart disease, COPD (lung diseases), cancers and dementia

Now it seems to me, and this is just *"Karl science"* here, **so please keep your quack-o-meter on high alert**, but maybe the sliding scale carries on up. Maybe instead of 5-a-day, we should be setting our sights on 7-a-day, as many scientists believe, or 10-a-day, or 15-a-day, or 20-a-day, because we might gain some benefits from those higher levels of nutrients. What do you think?

In some research studies, they have treated people with high-strength vitamin B3 therapy, and seen reductions in skin cancers.[12] They've taken kids with autistic spectrum disorders, and ADHD, and they have seen these

---

[12] Chen, A.C., Martin, A.J., Choy, B., et al (2015). A Phase 3 Randomized Trial of Nicotinamide for Skin-Cancer Chemoprevention. *N Engl J Med* 2015; 373:1618-1626. DOI: 10.1056/NEJMoa1506197

conditions improve by giving them B group supplements.[13] Same story with depression. If you show up in hospital with scurvy, they treat you with vitamin C, among other things. They treat anaemia with iron, and other supplements to help a person to absorb the iron. They can reverse beriberi by administering B1, and pellagra with B3. The point is this: taking vitamins and minerals away will kill you; putting them back in will fix things.

So, does it not seem logical that if B Group vitamins, calcium and iron, all help with energy production, red blood cells and muscular actions, and taking *below the RDA* of these things can leave you weak and lethargic, low on energy, below average...then *taking above the RDA of these things* just might help you have more energy, might help you to feel above average?

NOTE: Safe upper limits: There is an upper limit for a few of these micronutrients. For example, vitamin A is toxic at extreme amounts, and eating too much vitamin A all the time might be linked to some loss of bone mineral density in post-menopausal women, so I don't recommend eating liver twice daily, seven days per week. Selenium can become toxic at high amounts too, but in general, if your vitamins and minerals are coming from **whole foods**, not from supplement pills, and if you are eating a **sensible balanced diet** (hint: like *Mother Nature's Diet!!*) then you're very, **very** unlikely to ever eat too much of any vitamin or mineral.

Above the RDA

Now let's redraw our sliding scale graphic, going above that 'average' target as set by The Eatwell Plate, 5-a-day, and fish twice-per-week advice. I **speculate** that the secret to *better-than-average* immune system function, *better-than-average* energy production, *better-than-average* skin, hair, nails and eyesight, resisting the signs of ageing *better than the average person*, maybe the secret to all of this lies in a *higher-than-average* nutrient dense diet? Maybe there's a special 'awesome zone' up above the average line?

---

[13] Prousky, J.E. (2011). Vitamin Treatment of Hyperactivity in Children and Youth: Review of the Literature and Practical Treatment Recommendations. *Journal of Orthomolecular Medicine*, Vol 26 (3), 117-126. Retrieved from https://www.researchgate.net/publication/269929233_Vitamin_Treatment _of_Hyperactivity_in_Children_and_Youth_Review_of_the_Literature_and_Pra ctical_Treatment_Recommendations

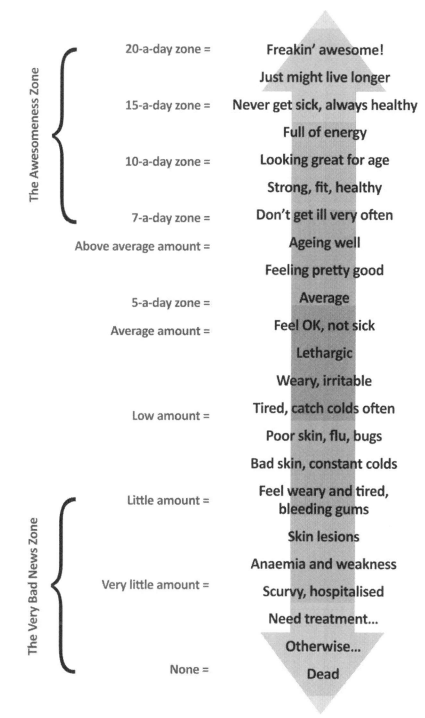

THE SLIDING SCALE

The Awesomeness Zone

20-a-day zone = Freakin' awesome!
Just might live longer
15-a-day zone = Never get sick, always healthy
Full of energy
10-a-day zone = Looking great for age
Strong, fit, healthy
7-a-day zone = Don't get ill very often
Above average amount = Ageing well
Feeling pretty good
5-a-day zone = Average
Average amount = Feel OK, not sick
Lethargic
Weary, irritable
Low amount = Tired, catch colds often
Poor skin, flu, bugs
Bad skin, constant colds
Little amount = Feel weary and tired, bleeding gums
Skin lesions
Anaemia and weakness
Very little amount = Scurvy, hospitalised
Need treatment...
Otherwise...
None = Dead

The Very Bad News Zone

People love to say to me, "But I'm not ill, I don't have a vitamin deficiency. I'm not wandering around being sick all the time, going to my doctor, and all that stuff."

And I will always reply "Yeah, you might not be ill, **but how much better could you be doing?** How much more energy could you have? How much better could you look for your age? How much more vitality could you be enjoying?"

- You say you want to resist the signs of ageing - I mean, no one actually *wants* to "look pretty shitty for 45" right?
- You say you want to resist minor illnesses - no one enjoys getting four or five coughs and colds every year
- You say you want more energy
- You say you want to feel good
- You say you want to resist chronic degenerative disease as you get older
- You say you want to look great, with gorgeous soft skin, shiny strong hair, shiny hard nails and bright healthy eyes
- You say you want good bowel and digestive function - because feeling bloated and farting isn't exactly a win for your sex life, right?
- You say you want to resist cognitive decline in older age
- You say you want to lose weight
- You say you want to look your best and feel self-confident

Everything you say you want from your health, I believe it's possible that the *Mother Nature's Diet* healthy lifestyle can provide it all. But we need to rise above this **'average thinking'** 5-a-day target. The abundant good health we are looking for, the *above-average* health and energy we seek lies in the 10-a-day zone, maybe in the 15-a-day zone, maybe in the 20-a-day zone!

From what I can tell, most of the general public get three or four coughs and colds per year, they complain they are sick and tired of feeling sick and tired, they **blame** everything from the weather, their boss and their spouse, to the government, 'airplane chemtrails' (don't get me started on that conspiracy quack nonsense) and the pharmaceutical companies. Folks are ageing badly, obesity, diabetes and cancer are on the rise, and most folks are ending up dying of heart disease or cancer a few years after retirement.

If that's even close to reality, if that's what we call 'average health' today, then I most certainly don't want to be average.

Ask yourself, if your health and your body are not looking too good from the outside, if you are ageing badly and your skin, hair, teeth, nails, eyes and energy levels are showing the signs outwardly, **what's happening on the inside? What can't you see?** Your skin is an organ. If that organ looks bad outside, then how are your other organs doing on the inside? Your heart, your brain, your liver? **That's something else there for you to ponder.**

Maybe I'm crazy, but…

I was that guy, I was Mr-below-average. I looked pretty shit for 18, pretty crap for 25, not great for 30, pretty out-of-shape for 35. I had skin problems, far less energy than I have now, bad breath, four of five coughs and colds per year and autoimmune issues (my nose and my skin). Then I cleaned up my lifestyle, improved my diet, formulated *Mother Nature's Diet* and became the 17-a-day guy.

Now I look pretty good for 48 (ha, ha, even if I say so myself!), I'm bursting with energy day and night, I never get sick, I have good skin, my medical issues have gone away and I feel great. Does that sound crazy to you?

Summary – what have we learned?

We've been through a lot of material in this chapter, let's summarise it in a few simple bullet points.

- Micronutrients, vitamins and minerals, are good for you, really good for you – without them, you die
- If you consume **below average** amounts of these nutrients, it's likely you will suffer **below average** health and ageing
- If you consume **above average** amounts of these nutrients, you just *might* enjoy **above average** health and ageing
- **I believe it all sits on a sliding scale – which means you can exert a fair bit of influence over where you sit on that scale**
- If you *choose* to eat a 2-a-day diet for life, avoid oily fish and liver, not get any exercise and little sunshine, you are likely to wallow down in the 'poor health' zone
- If you *choose* to eat a 12-a-day diet for life, eat fish five times per week, enjoy organ meats like liver from time to time, exercise daily, and get some fresh air and sunshine every day, you are likely to

enjoy living in the 'abundant good health' zone and look and feel great for your age

- Read those last three bullet points again, slowly, take it in
- Whaddya know – **you have a choice**
- I told you this book was trying to teach you three things, and one of them is that **you have more choice** over your health outcomes that you have been led to believe
- **You can control** (to some degree) how well you resist ill health, your immune function, how you resist the signs of ageing, how much energy you have, how you look and feel, and how likely you are to suffer degenerative disease as you grow older
- The answer is not to get your nutrients in supplement form. Studies show very little, or no, benefit to taking multivitamin and mineral pills[14] unless you have an illness or imbalance that needs treating. You want to eat real food, to consume these nutrients the way Mother Nature intended, in whole foods
- This chapter came after **Core Principle 1** for good reason. Remember in Core Principle 1, I encouraged you to replace those processed grains and starchy carbs with better foods? **Vegetables.** If you are going to start eating 12-a-day or 15-a-day, the only way to fit all that in, is to replace all that fattening starchy bulk with your extra veggies. That's why this part of the book is here, tagged on the end of Core Principle 1 – to get you moving towards 10-a-day and beyond

Wow, that chapter was huge. Well done for sticking with me. Now, take a stretch, grab a drink of water, and let's get back to the 12 Core Principles.

Rock on.

---

[14] Bjelakovic G, Nikolova D, Gluud LL, et al. (2012). *Antioxidant supplements for prevention of mortality in healthy participants and patients with various diseases.* Cochrane Review, 14 March 2012. Retrieved from https://goo.gl/Eaq8bk

Core Principle 2

U nless you have been avoiding all possible health and diet related articles in the press and on social media for the last five to ten years, then no doubt you have heard that 'sugar is the new fat', right? We are now facing the reality that the low-fat advice from the end of the 1970s to today has not served our population well! In the quest to remove fat from our diet, food manufacturers replaced the fat with more sugar, and the results have been disastrous. It seems it's sugar that's the major nutritional factor driving the obesity epidemic.

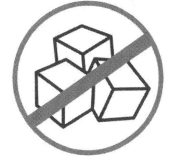

In 1965 in the UK, approximately 1.5% of the population were obese. It was considered a fairly rare medical condition. Now, half-a-century later, it's a **full third of our adult population**. Between 2014 and 2019, obesity rates around the UK stood between 28% and 30%. Additionally, **a further third** of our population are ranked as 'overweight'. Most worrying, childhood obesity is **rising even faster**. Health officials in the UK have declared rising obesity as one of the leading preventable causes of death in our country, and childhood obesity has been described, by the Health Secretary, as a "national emergency".

In round numbers, in half a century, we have gone from obesity being a minor condition, to one third of the population being obese, one third overweight, and only one third remaining at normal weight.

Pardon the unintended pun, but this is a *huge* problem, costing the UK economy many tens of billions per year in poor health and lost productivity, according to government statistics. Obesity is one of the major preventable contributing factors behind type-2 diabetes, heart disease, several common types of cancer and more.

Obesity, insulin resistance and type-2 diabetes

If you think the obesity epidemic is rising fast, the type-2 diabetes epidemic is rising twice as fast. There are now more than 3.8 million people in the UK with diabetes, that's around 10% of the entire adult population of the UK. According to figures sourced from the NHS [1], diabetes cost the UK approximately £23.7 billion (in 2010/11), including both direct and indirect costs. Approximately £9bn of that is direct costs for the NHS to treat type-2 diabetes, and an additional £13bn is indirect costs to the state, for premature deaths, loss of work and so on. The NHS further suggests that almost a million more people have type-2 diabetes and have not yet been diagnosed, and this is also already costing a further £1.5bn.

Worryingly, estimates suggest these figures are likely to almost double over the next 20 years. The rapid growth in type-2 diabetes is a worrying trend, yet in many cases the condition can be prevented, slowed, reversed or even cured, through changes to diet and lifestyle. Many would, and do, argue with this, but it remains a truth that large numbers of people have reversed and cured type-2 diabetes through diet and lifestyle changes. I have received many letters and emails from people telling me that they follow MND and they have eased or reversed their type-2 diabetes. At the very least, I strongly believe that in **many** cases type-2 diabetes can certainly be prevented from developing in the first place.[2]

Finally, ongoing research is looking at Alzheimer's Disease as a condition of insulin resistance in the brain. There are efforts to have Alzheimer's renamed to Type-3 diabetes.[3] Clearly, insulin resistance is a serious issue in this country. Type-2 diabetes is also a key marker for heart disease. Extensive evidence shows that a cluster of factors (commonly known as metabolic syndrome) including central obesity (abdominal fat), insulin resistance,

---

[1] NHS. (2012, April 25). *Diabetes: cases and costs predicted to rise.* Retrieved from https://www.nhs.uk/news/diabetes/diabetes-cases-and-costs-predicted-to-rise/

[2] NHS blog, (2018, April 19). *Type 2 diabetes and the importance of prevention.* Retrieved from https://www.england.nhs.uk/blog/type-2-diabetes-and-the-importance-of-prevention/

[3] See https://www.diabetes.co.uk/type3-diabetes.html

dyslipidaemia and high blood pressure, are key major risk factors for heart disease.[4]

It's becoming widely accepted[5] that excessive amounts of sugar and processed carbohydrates in our diet are major factors in these rising rates of obesity and insulin resistance. Excess dietary sugar (especially refined fructose) is a factor contributing to insulin resistance,[6] which in turn is exacerbating metabolic syndrome, various arthritic conditions, type-2 diabetes, heart disease, and more.

I meet people, almost every week, who tell me they've just been diagnosed with type-2 diabetes. All too often I find these people are pretty relaxed about the whole thing, they often just shrug it off with comments like "Oh well, I guess I've got to cut back on the cakes." This seems to me to be ignoring the seriousness of the condition. Being diagnosed type-2 diabetic takes around nine years off your life expectancy (depending on the individual, age and other risk factors), largely because diabetes is a major risk factor for heart disease, which is still the global number one killer. So, please don't be blasé thinking that being diagnosed diabetic just means, "Oh well, I can't have cake anymore." because it's actually a bit more serious than that.

Anecdotally, there are plenty of people from the UK, Europe, USA, Australia and New Zealand who follow *Mother Nature's Diet* for six months or a year, then email me saying "I'm off my meds, my type 2 diabetes has gone away." or "I've cured my chronic fatigue syndrome." or "My fibromyalgia is gone." or "My myofascial pain syndrome is gone." I know a handful of anecdotes does not make for a rigorous scientific study, but I receive emails from people in the USA saying, "My blood pressure's down. My diabetes is gone. I'm saving $400 per-month on the medications." All by following the 12 Core Principles of *Mother Nature's Diet*. Yes, these are just anecdotes, but I have received a lot of them. If you are suffering from high blood pressure, chronic fatigue syndrome or type-2 diabetes, don't you think it would be worth giving this healthy lifestyle a try?

---

[4] Laakso, M. (2010). Cardiovascular Disease in Type 2 Diabetes From Population to Man to Mechanisms. *Journal of Diabetes Care*, 2010 Feb; 33(2): 442–449. doi: 10.2337/dc09-0749

[5] See http://www.actiononsugar.org/sugar-and-health/

[6] *New theory on how insulin resistance, metabolic disease begin.* ScienceDaily online. (2016, Sept 26). Retrieved from https://www.sciencedaily.com/releases/2016/09/160926221442.htm

No miracle cure, no magic powder, just a year of cutting out the sugar and processed foods, exercising regularly, and eating a diet high in fresh whole foods. **I can't and never would** promise a 'cure all' for all people, and **legally I should remind you** that I am not a doctor and I can't promise to cure anyone of anything. But I can tell you **that anecdotally**, through email and social media, over the last few years I have received many such messages from people of all ages and in all situations, telling me that this lifestyle has helped them manage, reverse, or cure such health challenges.

Time to cut the sugar

In my opinion, as detailed above, eating too much refined sugar represents a major health challenge in the 21st century. Either in the form of the white crystals or cubes we know as table sugar, or in the liquid form used as a food additive, High Fructose Corn Syrup (HFCS), sugar is undeniably a major contributory factor to the rising global obesity and diabetes problem.

Food manufacturers seem to increasingly add sugar to almost every food, and some processed foods and soft drinks contain frightening amounts of refined sugar. With sugar added to everything from oven pizza to stir fry sauces, the problem is that people are becoming ever-more conditioned to expect all foods to taste sweet. This desire for sweet-tasting foods is a vicious cycle, driving over-eating of processed foods, and causing people to lose familiarity with the natural tastes of fresh whole foods.

Not a whole food

Refined sugar is not a nutritious food in and of itself, because it offers only calories, without any vitamins and minerals. Your body has to use small amounts of certain vitamins and minerals in order to process and metabolise refined sugar. Without getting all scientific on you, it requires a small amount of vitamin B1, B3, a little bit of vitamin C, a little bit of calcium, and a small amount of a few other minerals in order for you to metabolise the sugar you eat. By extension, therefore, it is technically an antinutrient,[7] something that costs your body micronutrients in return for the calories that it provides.

---

[7] Mother Nature's Diet blog. *White Refined Sugar is an Anti-nutrient.* (2014, Dec 23). See https://mothernaturesdiet.me/2014/12/23/white-refined-sugar-is-an-anti-nutrient/

If you lived on nothing but sugar, you would develop life-threatening vitamin deficiencies surprisingly quickly – scurvy, beriberi, pellagra and more.

In short, you would die faster eating a diet of just refined sugar, than if you ate nothing at all and slowly starved to death. Therefore, it's not an unrealistic notion to say that refined sugar is, technically, a mild poison.

Sugar: working against your 5-a-day

Framing refined sugar in this light, let's think about what that means for the average person's diet. As we saw in the previous chapter about micronutrients, while the government recommend 5-a-day, which may be setting the bar pretty damn low, the reality is that in fact two thirds of the nation don't eat their 5-d-a-day. **But what people do eat, is a lot of sugary foods and processed foods with refined sugar added.**

Let's look at some of those foods with lots of added sugar that most people eat on a daily basis:

- Breakfast cereal (loads of added sugar)
- Toast (added sugar, plus the toppings...jam, lemon curd, chocolate spread, marmalade, all loaded with sugar)
- Sliced white bread, filled bread roll, baguette or similar for lunch
- Evening meal – white pasta, white rice, spaghetti, etc.
- Snacks – biscuits, chocolate bars, cookies, cakes, donuts, bagels, pastries, sweets, etc.

Plenty of folks fill their days, and their bellies, with these foods, this is not uncommon. I meet people every week who eat these foods on a daily basis. They may also include some fruits and vegetables in their diet; typically, someone eating the foods listed above might also have one apple and one banana each day, and perhaps some limp salad in their baguette at lunch, and perhaps one or two servings of vegetables with their evening meal. So, they just about squeeze in 5-a-day if you use your imagination a bit!

But it's not just a case of saying, "Well, I eat my five a day, I have an apple, I have a banana, there was a lettuce leaf in my lunch and I have two veggies with my dinner, so there's my five a day. I'm good to go!" That's not enough,

if during the same day, they also consume five cups of tea with two sugars in each, a couple of cans of fizzy cola, a couple of chocolate chip cookies by the coffee machine mid-morning, two glasses of wine in the evening, and a chocolate bar or cake mid-afternoon. Combined with the breakfast cereal and the white bread sandwich, **this daily diet has a ton of sugar in it.**

From an obesity perspective, that person might get away with that diet if they are eating in caloric balance with a hefty training schedule, converting those sugary calories into exercise fuel. But from a micronutrients perspective, all that sugar is undoing the good of the vitamins and minerals in the 5-a-day. The sugar is an antinutrient, remember. So, the person who's eating this way isn't really getting his or her 5-a-day, because some of those vitamins and minerals are being used to metabolise all that sugar, so they are not ending up in his or her blood stream where they should be.

In reality, that person may be getting the fibre, and the calories, from their 5-a-day, but they are not getting the benefits of all those micronutrients. In terms of the vitamins and minerals, maybe they are only getting 3-a-day or 4-a-day, because of the losses to the antinutrient properties of the refined sugar.

I just made the exact numbers up, but I hope you understand the notion, that all the refined sugar is reducing the benefits of your 5-a-day, and remember, only a third of the population even eat their 5-a-day, which many scientists say is too low. I hope you can see that all this added sugar in our diet, is just further lowering the actual nutrient content of what we eat, driving our health down that 'sliding scale' we have been looking at.

Sugar addiction

Is sugar addictive? Does sugar 'stimulate the same pleasure centres in the brain as cocaine and an orgasm' as many reports in the media claim? Well, to be honest, the scientific jury is still out on that, some research shows in favour, and some shows that the effect is so small that such sensationalist headlines are a gross exaggeration.

But I see it this way – refined sugar is many, many times sweeter than anything Mother Nature makes available to us as a food source in the natural world. Perhaps honey is an exception to that statement, but realistically, in the natural world, how often and how widely available is honey? To our ancient 'caveman' ancestors, honey would have been a rare seasonal treat only available to those brave enough to climb rocks and trees to get it, facing swarms of angry bees defending the prize!

Because refined sugar is so sweet, it makes our food tastier, and promotes over-eating and emotional eating – comfort foods! Some people say that the obesity epidemic is a result of eating too much, and it's not the sugar driving obesity. Well, OK then, so maybe it's not the sugar itself promoting obesity, but the sweetness in modern processed foods that promote overeating – either way, sugar is a serious problem!

I don't think sugar is as chemically addictive as some narcotic drugs, or alcohol, but I do think that sweet tastes per se are addictive...even if that effect is more 'social crutch' than active biochemistry. In our wealthy Western culture, food has become a hobby, a pastime, a status symbol, an emotional back-stop, a go-to therapy, a leisure activity, an ecstatic experience, a boredom reliever, an anxiety drug, a time-filler and a way to fill the emotionally empty times in our lives when we fear feeling unfulfilled and alone. Nothing else but alcohol comes close to providing this social crutch, and sugar makes all the best comfort foods that much harder to resist.

Personally, it is my belief that the high levels of consumption of processed carbs (Core Principle 1) and refined sugar (Core Principle 2) are almost unquestionably **two of the key drivers behind the current obesity and type-2 diabetes epidemics.** Sugars are now hidden under an array of names and guises, some notorious like High-Fructose Corn Syrup (HFCS) and some more subtle, such as glucose-fructose syrup, or maltodextrin. Sugar is added to so many foods it is ridiculous – and often because the so-called 'food' is little more than 'nutritional cardboard' made in a factory, and without sugar it would taste pretty awful.

Feeling fruity

Core Principle 2 states 'Eliminate refined sugar. Limit natural sugars.' What do we mean by natural sugars? Largely, we are talking about fruit. Frustratingly, it's become somewhat fashionable in recent years for lean fitness trainer types to show off their 6-pack abs on YouTube or Instagram while telling people not to eat fruit, because it's "full of sugar and it'll make you fat".

Honestly, this bothers me. In a world where most people in Western society are eating far too much processed food, far too much processed carbohydrate and far too much refined sugar, warning people off a nutritious food group such as fruit seems like way the wrong message to me. In purposefully-brief bullet points, the truth goes roughly like this:

- Too much sugar is contributing to unwanted weight gain
- So, we need to cut back on sugar
- Fruit is full of a type of sugar, called fructose
- So, folks think they should cut back on fruit, to limit sugars
- Well, yes, but the human body metabolises fructose differently to how it metabolises other types of sugar, like the sugar we get from bread, pasta, or chocolate-chip cookies (which is sucrose or glucose)
- When we eat foods that provide glucose, the pancreas releases insulin, and this repeated insulin release is what's implicated in obesity and type-2 diabetes
- However, fructose does not stimulate the same insulin response that other sugars do, so fruit is actually OK!! Right?
- Well in fact, if you eat a lot of fruit, then the body takes what fructose it immediately needs, and then sends the excess to the liver for conversion into glucose anyway!
- That glucose then ends up stored as fat just like any other excess of glucose
- Doh! So, in fact, too much fruit will make us fat after all?
- Well, there are lots of good reasons to eat fruit, because it's a healthy natural whole food, meaning that fructose also comes packed with fibre, vitamins and minerals, and water, all of which are beneficial
- But, yes, an excessive amount of fruit at any one time may lead to an excess hit of sugar. If weight loss is your goal, then that 4-banana smoothie for breakfast probably isn't the best plan. Try scrambled eggs!

My oh my, you see how simple it all is!! Clear as mud, huh? You can see why we end up with these confusing videos on YouTube, with lean, muscular fit young people telling us to stay away from fruit! In reality, it's the fructose in added industrial syrups that is the big worry, not so much the fructose in fruit, unless you are diabetic or trying hard to lose excess weight.

I hope all this helps you to make sense of the fruit issue! If you hear anyone out there telling you, "you shouldn't eat fruit, fruit makes you fat" then that's a gross exaggeration and you cannot apply such advice on a 'one size fits all' basis for everyone. For a healthy person who is not particularly trying to lose weight, then eating an apple or an orange or some raspberries is all good, all part of a wonderful healthy diet. By contrast, someone grossly overweight trying to burn off those fat pounds, or a type-2 diabetic, might not be employing the best strategy if they are starting every day with a fruit smoothie and snacking on bananas twice daily.

I have met plenty of obese people who think a fruit smoothie is a good breakfast, and they love the sweeter fruits – banana, mango, grapes, papaya. For these people, 'cut back on your fruit' would be sound advice. Switching to a maximum of two servings of fruit per day, and focus on apples, citrus fruits or dark berries, might also be sound advice.

Selective breeding

It is also worth remembering that farmers have been practising a form of genetic modification for centuries called **selective breeding**. Through selective breeding, most fruits have become far bigger and sweeter today than they ever were in years gone by. 500 years ago, a banana was half the size, not so sweet, rather green and full of seeds. We have bred in those changes to make the big sweet yellow fruit we know today.

When we are learning about dietary approaches like the Paleo diet, it's important to remember that almost nothing on Earth is the same today as it was 100,000 years ago. Fruits, vegetables, animals, it's all changed. Maybe caveman ate several pieces of fruit per day, but it's important to realise that fruit back then, was different to the fruit we eat today.

Carbon footprint

It's also important to think about our carbon footprint when we are buying fruit. Here in the UK, we don't grow so many pineapples, bananas and coconuts. You know, I think it's got something to do with our weather...

The banana is the most popular fruit in the UK. All year round, we get through five bananas each, per person, per week, and it's important to remember that none of them are grown here, they are all imported from the tropics. That comes at a cost, and the environment is paying that price. Strawberries at Christmas. Coconut smoothies. Same deal. When it comes to buying fruit, maybe we should think seasonal, and think Fairtrade too. Let's be good global citizens.

Summary

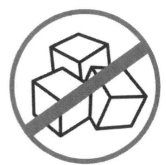

- Obesity and type-2 diabetes are on the rise in the UK, at an alarming rate
- Health officials in the UK have declared rising obesity as one of the leading preventable causes of death in our country, and childhood obesity has been described, by the Health Secretary, as a "national emergency"
- Sugar consumption is undeniably a major driver of the current rise in obesity, and a lot of research points to sugar consumption as one driver of the type-2 diabetes epidemic too
- Sugar is an antinutrient. Eating refined sugar actually does you more harm than good
- Refined sugar offers only empty calories, no vitamins and minerals. It costs your body small amounts of micronutrients to digest it
- If you tried to live on just refined sugar, you would almost certainly become very sick in surprisingly little time, and eventually die (faster than starving to death)
- Sugar is, therefore, technically, a mild poison
- Sugar could be described as 'emotionally addictive' and habit-forming, exacerbating over-eating and food addiction
- Many people think healthy fresh whole foods are boring, because they say they taste bland – but only to their palate which has been familiarised to desire sweet tastes by refined sugar and processed salt
- Sugar is in almost every processed food these days – study labels and wise up!
- Alcoholic drinks also contain a fair amount of sugar
- If you are trying to lose weight, cut back on the sweeter fruits, such as banana, papaya, mango and grapes
- Try to buy Fairtrade, and think about the carbon footprint of your fruit, and perhaps learn to shop more seasonally

Core Principle 3

Processed food. What do we mean by 'processed food'? I'm talking about everything from breakfast cereals, to frozen pizza. I'm talking about food from burger bars, fast-food joints, and take-away meals; those BBQ-flavoured crisps, snacks, and popcorn. I'm talking about jars and bottles of creams and sauces, microwave ready meals, sweets, crisps and noodles in a plastic pot. This covers fizzy drinks, energy drinks and confectionery. It pretty much covers almost everything edible they sell in convenience stores and petrol stations.

As far as I'm concerned, 90% or more of our diet should be made up of **fresh whole foods.** Everything else is processed. If it's got a label and a list of ingredients, and a bar code, and usually a picture on the front that says, 'Serving suggestion' then that's processed food. If the Use By date is much more than a week, then that's likely a processed food with added artificial preservatives.

Living the *Mother Nature's Diet* way, we want to avoid these processed foods as much as possible (and I appreciate that can be hard in our society these days) and eat almost exclusively fresh whole foods instead, rich in micronutrients and low in artificial additives.

Why?

Great question. I'm super glad you asked. This is another potentially vast topic, and this book is supposed to be an easy-going read, so there is not space to go into every sub-topic in great detail here. Instead, we'll just focus on a few key points in this book, and then if you want to learn more about all of these areas in detail, you can join our *MND Life!* community (see www.MotherNaturesDiet.com and 'Join the Club') or keep your eyes peeled for further books to follow this one.

I'll cover the following points as briefly as I can in this chapter:

- In Core Principle 1 we looked at removing the grains and starchy carbs from our diet, and in Core Principle 2 we looked at removing the refined sugar. Many processed foods contain both, so Core Principle 3 is helping you to live by CP 1 and 2
- Processed foods often lead to over-eating and hence contribute to weight gain
- Processed foods offer poor value-for-money compared to fresh whole foods. I'd rather pay for nutrients than packaging
- Everything about the processed food industry is wrong, in my opinion, it's not the direction we want to be heading in, it's the opposite of *Mother Nature's Diet*
- Nutrition, animal welfare and the dairy industry

First up then, Core Principle 3 is helping you stick to Core Principles 1 and 2. Let's explore this in a bit more detail. Many processed foods use the staples wheat, maize, soy, rice or potato as a base. Think pizza bases, breakfast cereals, pasta dishes, crisps and snacks and so on. The ingredients will often list wheat flour, potato starch, maize flour, rice flour or something similar as one of the first items listed in the ingredients list.

Do you know how ingredients lists work?
The first item listed is the thing that is most prevalent in that food, and then the second biggest item used is listed second, and so on. So, for the majority of foods, if you want to know what it is made of, just check out the first three or four items listed on the ingredients list, and that probably accounts for 95% to 98% or more of that food by weight, or by calories, then all the rest are the minor ingredients, such as added preservatives, colourings, flavours, emulsifiers and so on.

For a great majority of processed foods, you'll find those first few ingredients tend to be some kind of grain, flour or starch, and then added sugar. These foods almost always include sugar and salt, because, frankly, they taste like shit without them.

Think about it: they've taken some kind of wheat or rice starch, refined it, processed it and denatured it so that it won't go rancid or rotten. This extends its shelf life, and then they have beaten and bashed it into whatever shape or form they require. Then it has preservatives and colourings added. By this point, in my opinion, it's little more than 'nutritional cardboard' in both nutrition value and taste.

Does that sound like an exaggeration? **Could this be quackery I am sharing?**

Well in the UK (and most other countries too) it's illegal to sell any wheat flour that has not been fortified. All flour for bread making or pasta manufacture, has to be fortified, by law[1], with nutrients such as vitamin B1 and iron. Why do you suppose that is?

Maybe you remember growing up with Kellogg's cereals, back in the 1970s and 80s, they always had that big red 'corner slash' triangle on the front of the packet stating, "Fortified with vitamins and minerals" – why? Because flour, bread, cereals and pasta, would contain almost no micronutrients at all if they didn't.

Processed foods tend to be made from a base of some kind of bleached, refined starch, fortified artificially to give it some nutritional value, and then they add sugar to make it taste nice. They usually add salt and often processed vegetable oils, or palm oil, to add substance and flavour. That's usually it, the majority of the food is made of these basics, and then the last few percent are all the flavourings and colourings added to distinguish one 'food product' from another.

The illusion of choice

You can look in a large British supermarket and find 80,000 different product lines. Maybe 50,000 food items to choose from. This is the **illusion of choice**. The bright colours, the eye-catching packaging, the names and pictures, the range of delicious flavours – 70 or 80 or 90 types of breakfast cereal, a dozen choices of ketchup, 30 or 40 flavours of ice cream, 20 types of frozen pizza. This is the illusion of choice – 50,000 shapes, colours and flavours, but

---

[1] *The Bread and Flour Regulations 1998.* (1998). Schedule 1. Essential Ingredients of Flour. Retrieved from http://www.legislation.gov.uk/uksi/1998/141/schedule/1/made

underneath a selection of artificial chemical flavours and colours, it's the same dozen basic ingredients in everything.

Massive variety of choices to stimulate your mind and senses and encourage you to spend more money, **but virtually no biodiversity in terms of nutrition.** This is the world of processed food: it's all about calories, not nutrition. Let's check out a few food labels and see what I am talking about.

Food labels

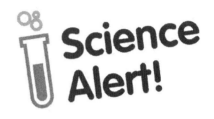

A carrot does not have a label saying, "Ingredients: 100% carrot". When you visit a proper butcher, and ask for a shoulder of lamb, it does not come with a label with a list of ingredients, a bar code and a pretty picture of sunrise over an old farm house. It comes out of the cool room at the back with blood smeared on it and likely some bones poking out. The butcher may saw any excess bone off for you, then he weighs it and wraps it in a piece of paper and you take it home. That is real food. Fresh food. Whole food. That is how it should be.

By contrast, let's look at some randomly-picked processed food products to see what they are really made of (and I am just copying text from the ingredients labels here, 100% verbatim at time of writing):

Ingredients label 1 – Bisto Best Rich & Roasted Pork Gravy granules: Potato Starch; Dried Glucose Syrup; Salt; Flavourings (Contains Milk); Flavour Enhancers (E621, E635); Vegetable Oil; Colour (E150c); Dried Pork (0.4%); Emulsifiers (Soya Lecithin); Onion Extract; Rosemary Extract.

What do we see here? Potato starch (there it is, #1 biggest ingredient, a cheap processed starch), #2 ingredient, dried glucose syrup (sugar, basically), salt, then minor additives. You can see that by the time we get down to 'dried pork' on the ingredients list, we are down to 0.4% of the food. That means that the items on the list before the dried pork, account for over 99% of the food's make-up by weight.

That first example completely and perfectly makes the point. Gravy granules, they are basically made of processed starch with added sugar and salt, then some artificial flavours, colours and preservatives. That's it.

Let's try another. And please know that I really just picked these items pretty much at random, I have not gone out of my way to pick 'bad' examples for you. If I wanted to do that, these examples would all be oven pizza, ice cream, microwave popcorn and chocolate chip cookies. You don't have to believe me if you don't want to, feel free to randomly pick some processed foods yourself and work through the ingredients lists understanding what they are made of.

Ingredients label 2 – Sharwood's Medium Egg Noodles: Wheat Flour; Egg (5.5%); Salt; Acidity Regulator: Potassium Carbonate.

And now we see a very similar story again in egg noodles, which are mainly (about 93% to 94% I would estimate) made of wheat flour, then egg and salt. Well, at least it doesn't have a bunch of added sugar! Let's look at another.

Ingredients label 3 – Whole Earth Lightly Whipped Milk Chocolate Spread: Sugar; Palm Oil; Lactose; Low Fat Cocoa Powder (10%); Skimmed Milk Powder; Whey Powder; Emulsifier: Soya Lecithin; Flavouring: Bourbon Vanilla Extract.

The number one item on the list is sugar, then palm oil which has been the target of massive press attention because of deforestation and loss of habitat for orangutans (more on that coming up). Ingredient number three is lactose, that's milk sugar, followed by cocoa powder and skimmed milk powder, whey powder and then the emulsifier and flavourings. This product, sold under the Whole Earth brand, is made from a boat-load of sugar, some skimmed milk powder and palm oil. Bad for you and bad for the environment. What the heck is supposed to be so healthy and wholesome about that? Yet the 'Whole Earth' brand is all 'pictures of trees' and green lettering, like we are somehow supposed to think it's environmentally friendly, and maybe good for us. It's just a jar of sugar and oil. OK, to our last example:

Ingredients label 4 – Kellogg's Crunchy Nut with red fruit bites: Cereals (Oats, Maize); Sugar; Vegetable Oil; Crisp Cereal (Rice Flour, Maize Flour, Sugar, Skimmed Milk Powder, Salt, Dextrose); Glucose Syrup; Raspberry Flavour Fruit Pieces (6%) (Sugar, Cranberry, Citric Acid, Flavouring, Elderberry Juice From Concentrate); Peanuts (4.5%); Strawberry Fruit Pieces (3%) (Fructose-Glucose Syrup, Humectant {Glycerol}, Sugar, Strawberry Puree from Concentrate, Oat Fibre,

Vegetable Oil, Rice Starch, Gelling Agent {Pectin}, Vegetable Concentrate {Pumpkin, Carrot}); Modified Starch; Salt; Barley Malt Flavouring; Sodium Bicarbonate; Antioxidant (Ascorbyl Palmitate, Alpha Tocopherol); Emulsifier (Soy Lecithin).

And breakfast cereals here provide another perfect example – ingredients in order of weight are highly processed grains, a bunch of sugar, some oils, and then a heap of artificial additives to try to make it taste and look nice. Please note that any brand names mentioned are just examples, I am not picking on these food manufacturers in particular, most other manufacturers are just the same.

Four examples, from seemingly very diverse food products – gravy granules, egg noodles, chocolate spread and breakfast cereal – yet they are actually all made from roughly the same stuff. Some grain or starch, highly denatured and processed, add sugar, add refined oil, add salt, add artificial colours and flavours. **That's the illusion of choice.**

Lots of colours and flavours…just bugger all nutrition

What all these products show is that most processed foods are made of the same handful of staple food products – wheat, rice starch, potato starch, sugar, corn starch and so on. Our supermarkets today create the illusion of choice, the illusion of plenty, but the reality is that these 'food products' offer very little nutritional biodiversity.

Additionally –

- Many processed foods contain excess cheap processed refined salt, more than most people need (especially people who might have high blood pressure)
- They often contain refined vegetable/seed oils, which can be adding undesirable and potentially harmful fats to your diet
- They often contain palm oil – more on that coming up
- Processed meats, such as these formed lunch meats, packets of ham shaped like dinosaurs and so on, and most cheap meat products (snacking sausages and similar) contain sodium nitrite and other preservatives that have been questioned as possible carcinogens. The cheap processed meat market will be covered in more detail later, under Core Principle 8

Processed food, 'food addiction' and over-eating

These are all vast topics, I think I could write a whole book just on Core Principle 3! But I am trying to keep all this as brief and simple as I can for you, while still explaining enough to make my points, to help you understand the rationale behind each of the 12 Core Principles and how your health will benefit from following this lifestyle.

One of the problems with processed foods is that they often encourage over-eating, and this is a major factor in driving the current rise in obesity. Think about our ancient ancestors, those hunter-gatherers who lived ten, twenty, fifty thousand years ago. Our genes evolved back then, living the way they lived, and although I wasn't alive fifty thousand years ago so I can't say for sure, I have read a lot of books on genetics, evolution, anthropology and history, and I am pretty certain that Pizza Hut and Ben & Jerry's ice cream weren't around back in the Paleolithic era.

These modern foods are extremely tasty, they 'tick all our boxes' when we eat them (I will explain why) and we just want more. They have turned eating into a pleasurable activity in a way that our caveman ancestors can never have known, and our brains **simply don't know how to stop wanting them.** We are genetically predisposed to over-eat, we are genetically wired to just want more, and it's incredibly difficult to say no, to stop when we have had enough.

Food manufacturers know this, and in fact they purposefully manufacture foods that are formulated to hit something called your 'bliss point'.[2] When they make a new pasta sauce or a new tomato soup, or a new cereal, or a new type of pizza, or whatever it might be, they'll create the general shape and colour of the product, get the texture right, then get the exact flavour that they want. They'll make about 40 or 50 different versions of each food with minutely different adjusted amounts of salt, fat, and sugar and then they set up tests with panels of volunteer tasters, to find out precisely which flavour just hits that perfect spot – the spot where you just can't get enough!

---

[2] Reading for further interest on this fascinating topic: *The Extraordinary Science of Addictive Junk Food.* New York Times Magazine. (2013, Feb 20). Retrieved from https://www.nytimes.com/2013/02/24/magazine/the-extraordinary-science-of-junk-food.html

This is how they create something called **hyperpalatable foods**. To you and I, they are called *irresistible*, or *delicious*, or *utterly moreish*, or *soooo yummy*! If you're interested in learning more about this, just search for 'hyperpalatable foods' and 'bliss point' online and read about the science of how they're making you buy more food than you need or even want.[3] They're making you fat and driving up obesity by making food that's quick and easy to heat, easy to cook, easy to eat, easy to chew, easy to digest, **and you just want more of it.** Then you wonder why you're lethargic and got bad skin, you're overweight and you feel like crap. That's another big reason why we want to take the processed foods out of our diet.

High in calories, low in nutrients

As we have seen, most processed foods are made from a base of some grain or starch, with added sugar. This means that these foods, when compared to fresh whole foods, tend to be high in calories, but low in nutrients. These highly processed foods might appear to be cheap, for the number of calories you are getting. But if we measured their content by beneficial nutrients instead, we would see that they are actually not cheap at all.[4]

Value for money – *your* money

At the start of this chapter, I listed five reasons why we want to ditch the processed foods from our diet. The third reason listed was because processed foods offer poor value-for-money compared to fresh whole foods. I'd rather pay for nutrients than packaging. Let's look at this now. This is the last big one, hang in there, you're doing great!

When you go shopping in a British supermarket and you fill your trolley up, for the sake of simplicity in this example, let's say there's about £100 of shopping in a full trolley. The real food, the stuff that comes from a farm, this is **plants and animals** (Core Principle 7), the meat, the fish, the vegetables,

---

[3] Of interest on this topic, check out the brilliant Malcolm Gladwell TED talk *Choice, happiness and spaghetti sauce*, from Feb 2004, available here https://www.ted.com/talks/malcolm_gladwell_on_spaghetti_sauce
[4] Mother Nature's Diet blog. *Why we have an obesity problem Part #2.* (2019, Feb 7). See https://mothernaturesdiet.me/2019/02/07/why-we-have-an-obesity-problem-part-2/

the fruits, accounts for about £20 of the money you spend. These are *average* figures for the whole UK, averaged over recent years – of all the money Brits spend annually on buying food in supermarkets, approximately 20% of that money goes to farmers. (In the United States, it's much less, only half as much.)

Out of that £100, you are spending £20 to buy actual food. The rest, the other £80, you're paying Mondelēz International, Nestle, PepsiCo, Heinz and Unilever, and all the other big food companies to beat it, shape it, colour it, flavour it, heat it, treat it, turn spaghetti into alphabet shapes, preserve it, label it, make dinosaur shaped chicken pieces, name it, package it and freeze it. And of course, you're paying the supermarkets to drive the stuff around the country and get it all on the shelves for you.

When you spend £100 in a typical British supermarket, filling your trolley with a range of food products from across the store, you're only actually spending £20 on the proteins, the vitamins, the minerals, the fats, the carbohydrates, the food, the nutrients. The other £80, you're paying for the shaping, colouring, processing and packaging; you're paying for the radio and TV advertising campaigns, magazine advertising, the promotions, the toy in the breakfast cereal, the competition coupon on the box, the frozen warehousing, the distribution, the supermarket shelves, and so on.

Please just think about that
for a few moments.

I'm going to explain this in more detail **over the next four pages** – if you don't care much about the politics and economics of food, then go ahead and skip these pages, it's fine. However, if you want to know why our modern food supply is messed up, then please read on.

Spend on nutrition, not packaging

If I spend £100 in the supermarket, and only £20 ends up going back to the farmer, perhaps (guesswork on my part) another £20 pays for the additives, processing, colouring, preserving, freezing, shaping and flavouring. Now I have spent £40 on food, half of which paid for the actual raw materials – the meat, fish and plants. This raises two questions:

1. How have I got a whole trolley full of food, **and this actual food only cost £20?** When I go to the local farm shop and buy organic meat and organic vegetables grown within a few miles of my house, a similar sized trolley full of food would cost at least £200! Ten times as much. How can the actual food part of my supermarket spend be so low?
2. Where did the other £60 go?

Let's break these questions down and understand what people are spending their money on.

I'm making some broad sweeping assumptions here, and using rough round numbers that are approximately right (at time of writing), but hopefully you will agree that I am not far off. If I go to my local supermarket (I have a Sainsbury's, a Morrison's, three Tesco's, an M&S Food Hall, a Co-op, a Lidl and an Aldi to choose from in the town where I live) and fill a regular trolley to near-full, what you might call a 'level load' including a little fresh meat such as a joint for Sunday roast, some fruits and vegetables, such as apples, potatoes, carrots, bananas, and then all the usual things a normal family buys every week – cereals, bread, pasta, stir-in sauces, several pints of milk, an oven pizza, some oven chips, some crisps, biscuits, soft drinks, jam and so on. I'm leaving expensive alcohol out of this for now. From my experience, allowing for price variety in different shops around different parts of the country, this trolley full of food will likely cost around £100.

By contrast, if I go to my local farm shop and buy only fresh whole foods – foods that use zero packaging except the paper bags I put them in when I purchase them, or the piece of wrapping the butcher puts around a fresh joint of meat when I select it over the counter – then a similar sized 'level load' in a similar sized trolley, will almost certainly cost in excess of £200.

This trolley full of food will likely include fresh joints of lamb, beef or pork, possibly wild local game if it's available, and fresh chicken; locally grown seasonal vegetables, some fruits, and some locally made organic dairy such as cheese or yoghurt.

At the local farm shop, I will assume that 10% of my bill is profit, and 20% of that bill is overheads for running and staffing the shop, its lights, refrigerators, cash registers, credit card machines and so on. That means I have paid around £140 for the actual food (plus farm staff, farm running costs, butcher, etc.). This is real food – the vegetables still have some mud on them. The fruits have imperfections. The meat is bloody and does not come shrink wrapped in plastic with a polystyrene tray and a barcode on it. I can watch my butcher working out back behind the counter, cutting up an entire pig into joints. He will often cut a joint to order for me, to the size and weight I ask for.

When I visit the farm shop, I spend £140 (out of £200 total spend) on fresh, nutritious whole foods (and 'food production') and take home enough food to feed my family for a week. It's additionally cost me £60 to pay for the convenience of shopping there, and I know the carbon footprint of my food is lower, as it is all locally produced, at most within a 'two country' radius, but no international imports.

Compare the above example to the supermarket: I have £20 worth of real food, approximately £20 spent on processing that food (my estimate), and then the other £60 covers:

- Packaging, the cardboard, polystyrene and plastic, the printing and the barcode
- Refrigerated transport, fuel (and the pollution that goes with it)
- Warehousing and storage
- The overhead of the supermarket
- The print and TV advertising that is used to promote and sell these foods, such as breakfast cereals, frozen pizza, soft drinks and ice cream brands
- The profit for the food manufacturer, profit for the refrigerated transport company, profit for the supermarket

None of these things are foods or nutrients.

None of these things are measurable in nutrient value. A TV ad campaign for a certain make of oven chips **won't help my child to have more energy.** An annual bonus for the truck driver or his company bosses won't make my immune system function any better. Supermarket shelves [5] organised in ways[6] to promote 'product discovery'[7] (purposefully make me buy more stuff I didn't know I wanted in the first place) won't ensure I'm getting plenty of minerals and eating high quality omega-3 fats every day. **These things don't provide me with any nutrient value, but I am paying for them just the same.**

When we shop in the supermarket and buy predominantly processed foods, that's what we are paying for. We're paying to run the food industry, rather than paying for nutrition.

Now you might say: "But Karl, you could go to the supermarket, spend £100 and feed your family for a week, or go to the farm shop and spend £200+ to feed your family for a week. Why pay twice as much? Looking at your rough calculations above, *it seems the food manufacturers and supermarkets are doing us all a great favour, through economies of scale, they have driven food prices right down.* Isn't that a good thing?"

Let's see. Here's the reality. Those prices that are driven down so low...

- That's why farm animals are mistreated and often live in dirty, inhumane conditions. Chickens in cages. Pigs behind bars. Cows that live in barns and never go outside to range freely on grass
- That's why small family farmers go broke and have to sell their farms to big industrial operations, because they are driven down so hard on food prices – to pay for that printed cardboard packaging, and that TV ad campaign, and that refrigerated warehousing

---

[5] Chen, Y., Chen, J. & Tung, C. (2006). A data mining approach for retail knowledge discovery with consideration of the effect of shelf-space adjacency on sales. *Elsevier: Decision Support Systems*, 42(3), 1503-1520. https://doi.org/10.1016/j.dss.2005.12.004

[6] Aloysius, G., & Binu, D. (2012). An approach to products placement in supermarkets using PrefixSpan algorithm. *Journal of King Saud University - Computer and Information Sciences*, 25(1), 77-87. https://doi.org/10.1016/j.jksuci.2012.07.001

[7] *The science that makes us spend more in supermarkets, and feel good while we do it.* (2014, March 5). Retrieved from https://phys.org/news/2014-03-science-supermarkets-good.html

- That's why croplands are sprayed with chemicals, degrading the soil, polluting local rivers, killing fish and eroding away topsoil
- That's why vegetables have a lower nutritional value (fewer minerals) today than they had 50 years ago, because the soils are depleted from constant use, in the name of profit
- That's why so many farmers in the UK are working at a loss, and struggling to stay in business, while the big food companies make billions in profits
- That's why fruits and vegetables imported from the tropics carry a heavy carbon footprint, a cost that the environment is paying
- That's why overseas farmers in far flung developing markets are suffering human rights abuses and struggling to survive (Hint: buy Fairtrade)
- That's why many dairy cows are mistreated and after only three years 'in service' they are exhausted and are no longer fit for milking
- That's why rainforests in the Far East are being cut down to grow palm oil to make processed foods taste nicer, so that we buy more, even though the Sumatran tiger [8] and the orangutan [9] both face imminent extinction

The ugly reality is that your food shop is cheap because the money that should be used to pay our farmers to be responsible stewards of the land, to nurture and nourish our arable soils, to protect trees and hedgerows, to treat animals kindly and with respect, to ensure slaughter is a clean, minimally-painful, quick operation; this money is instead spent on adding sugar and flavour enhancers to your food to make it tastier, so you buy more, and on advertising campaigns and marketing tricks that are driving the obesity epidemic by encouraging people to overeat these hyperpalatable foods.

These are the true costs of cheap food. That's how the big food manufacturers, distributors and supermarkets deliver at such low prices for those 'food products' in your trolley.

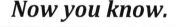

Now you know.

[8] See https://www.onegreenplanet.org/environment/how-palm-oil-impacts-the-sumatran-tiger/
[9] See https://orangutan.org/rainforest/the-effects-of-palm-oil/

Mother Nature's Diet is different

So far in this chapter, you have learned that –

- Many processed foods are just made of some kind of flour or starch, with sugar and salt added, then artificial colours and flavourings to differentiate the various foods from each other – this is the illusion of choice
- Manufacturers add sugar, salt and fats/oils to food to make them hyperpalatable, driving over-eating and obesity. Humans are genetically predisposed to overeat when faced with this endless tide of sweet, delicious food
- 80% of the money you spend in a supermarket goes on things that don't provide you with any actual nourishment
- The illusion of cheap food comes at a price – a price paid by mistreated animals, hard-working farmers, the environment, and your health

Processed foods are the output of the industrialised food system – that is the food product wholesalers and distributors, the big food manufacturers, the distributors and supermarkets. Big Food and Big Ag as some call them. Living the *Mother Nature's Diet* way, we aim to stop supporting the industrialised food system...**by not giving them our money!** The best way to cast a vote against the system is to spend your money elsewhere.

At this point, Sam Walton, the famous founder of Walmart stores, seems an odd man to quote (he is clearly one of the kings of supermarket retail!) but this line is worth remembering –

"There is only one boss. The customer. And he can fire everybody in the company from the chairman on down, simply by spending his money somewhere else."

Remember – you're the boss. If you read the previous four pages and you didn't like what you saw, you can vote for change by spending your money elsewhere. The more of us take our money away from the industrialised food system, the more our voices will be heard.

Vote for change by –

- Shopping at local farm shops and farmer's markets
- Use local independent butchers, fishmongers, green grocers
- Build a relationship with your butcher, ask where the food comes from, how the animals were fed, what conditions they lived in. Be interested
- Pay attention. Learn. Care
- Buy Fairtrade
- Buy organic
- Buy free range. Buy pasture raised or grass-fed
- Find a local farm selling free range eggs direct to the public
- Plant up a few square feet in your garden and try growing some of your own food
- Eat seasonally – remember the carbon footprint of those strawberries in winter

There are many ways you can change your shopping habits to stop supporting the industrialised food system and start supporting small 'local food webs' instead. People sometimes say to me, "Oh, I can't afford your elitist diet. I can't afford to go to the farm shop and buy all that organic food."

It's a fair point, but at least when you go to your local farm shop and pay £40 for a big joint of beef or something, at least you're giving your £40 to the farmer, not the food company. (And as an aside…you **can** afford it. Take your alcohol and confectionery budget, and spend it on real food instead!) **Pound for pound**, I'll bet your family gets *more nutrients from the farm shop* than they do from the supermarket. Not just calories – actual beneficial nutrients.

Ask yourself, do you want to pay for calories, or do you want to pay for nutrition?

Something else to think about there.

Cruelty in dairy

And so to the last point, and I promise to keep this brief, as I know this chapter has turned out to be huge, and you need to take a breather. Core Principle 3 states 'only eat organic, raw, or grass-fed dairy'. This again could fill an entire book on its own (yawn, sorry I keep saying that!), but the basic message is this –

There's milk, and there's milk.

All milk is not the same! Let's unpack this and see what it means. If a cow lives her life eating grains and corn, stuck in a barn, miserable, pregnant, exhausted and unhealthy, then she's going to produce milk with different nutritional values to the milk from a cow that lives her life outside on pasture, eating grass, healthier, less stressed and less exhausted. One way is bad for the cow, and less nutritious for us. The other way is a good life for the cow, and makes better food for us. That's frustratingly brief and missing a lot of detail, but that's the argument in a nutshell. Core Principle 8 will expand on this slightly adding that the grass-fed organic cow is better for the environment too.

There is a lot of cruelty in the dairy industry. I think it's fair to say that there is more cruelty in the average pint of milk than there is in the average pound of beef (I wish I could remember who first said that line and give them credit for it.). So, if you want to make a stand for better standards in animal welfare, one good step in the right direction is to buy organic milk, and ideally, 100% grass-fed milk. You'll be buying a nutritionally superior food, and you'll be helping to take the cruelty out of dairy farming.

Living and eating the MND way, we avoid all mass-market pasteurised milk and cheese, so if the regular, cheap, 'supermarket stuff' is your only option, then it's best just to drop it altogether. But if you are prepared to stretch your budget to the organic options, then we can enjoy a little dairy in our diet.

- Grass-fed butter for cooking scrambled eggs (my local Sainsbury's stocks grass-fed unpasteurised butter) or organic goat's butter
- Personally, I buy goat's milk yoghurt for use as a condiment. Feta cheese is good too (goat's cheese)
- A little organic artisanal cheese goes a long way to liven up a salad

- There are some good healthy cheese options available - Parmigiano Reggiano is grass-fed and unpasteurised, and man those cows are looked after well, and French Comté is also excellent
- A pot of organic heavy cream from a local farm makes a treat from time to time

There is far more to it than this, but this book is only meant to be a brief study of the topic, so if you want to know more and learn all the details, then do please visit *Mother Nature's Diet* dotcom and join us in the **MND Life! community** or keep your eyes peeled for a much more detailed book in the future.

Phew!! That was a big chapter with a lot of material to cover. We made it!!! Hoorah! Well done you!

Summary

Core Principle 3: Minimise processed foods, eat only organic raw or grass-fed dairy. It's taken 14 pages to cover this, and as the writer I feel I have barely scratched the surface of these many complex and inter-related topics! Here are the key take-away points; the main reasons we want to minimise the amount of processed foods in our diet:

- Processed foods are mostly made of grains and sugar
- The illusion of choice
- Nutritionally, these foods are vastly inferior to fresh whole foods
- Hyperpalatable foods add sugar, salt and fats to find your bliss point, to encourage you to overeat
- Our genetic tendency to pig out when it's available, make these foods damned hard to resist
- It's all adding to the obesity problem
- The easiest way to avoid eating these foods – don't buy them! If they are not in your home, that's a big help
- 80% of the money you spend in a supermarket goes on things that don't provide you with any actual nourishment. Advertising,

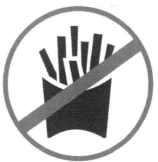

colourings and flavourings, toys in the cereal box, packaging, warehousing, distribution, point-of-sale material, etc.
- Readers in the United States - same, but worse, your farmers get even less than the 20% farmers here in Europe are getting
- Spend your money with farmers whenever possible – the fewer steps between farmer and consumer, generally speaking, the better
- Better for the farmer, better for you, usually better for the soil and the farm animals
- The illusion of cheap food comes at a price – a price paid by mistreated animals, hard-working farmers, the environment, and your health
- Mainstream pasteurised dairy, the mass-market stuff in the supermarkets, is nutritionally weak and comes with animal welfare concerns
- Avoid processed foods! Base 90% or more of your diet on fresh, nourishing, whole foods

Core Principle 3 - done! Phew! Take a break, go stretch your legs, have an apple, drink a glass of water, you deserve to give your eyes and brain a rest! Well done for getting through that! I promise you, Core Principles 1 and 3 are "the biggies" and things should all get a bit easier now and the next few Core Principles should flow a bit faster for you.

Core Principle 4

There is some common, and some not-so-common sense in Core Principle 4. There are some pretty obvious good health tips here, like quitting smoking, but then we also have to tackle some 'less popular' topics, like the fact that far too many people are drinking far too much alcohol. We also need to look at the total load of chemicals in our lives.

Smoking

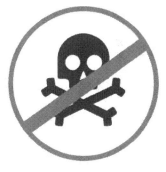

Don't smoke. Really, we all understand that already, don't we? Smoking is the leading preventable cause of death worldwide, and smoking kills around 6.5 million people around the world every year. Smoking is the cause behind approximately 80,000 deaths in the UK every year, or one in every six, including around 23% of cancer deaths annually. 12% of all new cancer cases in the UK are caused by smoking. It is our leading preventable cause of death and our leading preventable cause of cancer, and we have known this now for decades, it's not like this is coming to anyone as new information.

It's on the NHS's website; it's on Cancer Research UK's website; it's on the British Heart Foundation's website, and many more. Every site offers major tips on prevention – how to prevent cancer, how to prevent heart disease. **Tip number one: don't smoke.** If you smoke and need to quit, get some help. I know how it is, I smoked for 20 years. I say go and see your doctor, he or she can give you patches, or gum, or put you in touch with a clinic to help. The NHS has a proven, effective smoking cessation programme. It's free, they're there waiting to help you, as a taxpayer you're paying for it, so go get it, go get that help, it works.

It says on every pack, 'this may kill you'.
Please don't smoke, it's stupid, just don't do it.

Alcohol

If food is the world's most widely-used emotional crutch, then alcohol is surely the world's most widely-used anxiety drug. Addressing the topic of alcohol consumption is a big deal for a lot of people.

Giving up alcohol, or cutting right back, can be a tough thing to do, because many people (in my experience) don't realise that they are drinking too much and it's not good for their health. Alcohol has a lot of known negative health consequences; it contributes to some 200 health conditions[1], including obesity, sexual dysfunction, liver disease, breast and bowel cancer, depression and degenerative neurological conditions. According to Cancer Research UK[2], 4% of all cancer in the UK is directly attributable to drinking alcohol, **making it the fourth leading preventable cause of cancer in the UK.** Drinking alcohol contributes to seven types of cancer, including breast cancer, and can lead to liver damage and liver disease.

The government changed their guideline advice on tolerable alcohol limits at the tail-end of 2015, when the Chief Medical Officer said, "Drinking any level of alcohol carries a risk." The folks at Cancer Research UK also say, "There's no 'safe' limit for alcohol when it comes to cancer, but the risk is smaller for people who drink within the government guidelines."

According to PHE, Public Health England:
In England, 10.4 million people [note: that's a quarter of the adult population] consume alcohol at levels above the UK Chief Medical Officers' low-risk guideline and increase their risk of alcohol-related ill health.

The economic burden of alcohol is estimated between 1.3% and 2.7% of annual GDP.

---

[1] PHE. *Health Matters: preventing ill health from alcohol and tobacco use.* (2017, October 4). Retrieved from https://www.gov.uk/government/publications/health-matters-preventing-ill-health-from-alcohol-and-tobacco/health-matters-preventing-ill-health-from-alcohol-and-tobacco-use
[2] Learn more https://www.cancerresearchuk.org/about-cancer/causes-of-cancer/alcohol-and-cancer/does-alcohol-cause-cancer

Every unit carries a risk. So, how much is safe for you to drink? Well, how much do you want to reduce your cancer risk? **You choose, you decide.** Your health is in your hands. See, again, **you have a choice.** The less you drink, the more you reduce cancer risk.

Beyond its role as society's #1 drug of choice, the risk of addiction, and the increased risk of various chronic diseases as listed above, alcohol further adds additional calories to your diet, and – in my opinion – clouds your mind and slowly drains your mental faculties. [Though, on that point, once again we note that once size does not fit all. Some people handle alcohol very well, some don't. It can be due to genetic nuances, and there are other factors involved too.]

Is the beer making me fat?
The short answer is, 'yes, probably.'

Alcoholic drinks are pretty high in calories and heavy drinking will almost certainly contribute to weight gain, particularly fat weight. I read the other day that "a large glass of wine per day adds up over the week to more than 1500 calories per week – it's like eating a Cornetto every day!" That's just one glass of wine per evening.

Your relationship with alcohol

Personally, I am teetotal; I haven't had a drink for over seven years and three months now, at time of writing. When I did drink, I was never very good at regulating it. When I used to drink, I used to like to drink every day, often a fair bit. For 26 years, I had what I would describe as a moderately unhealthy relationship with alcohol. For me, I can put my hand on my heart and say, that being teetotal, "It's the single best thing I've ever done for my own health." I would sooner start smoking again than drinking, I feel that strongly about it. Quitting is a pretty big deal for many people. It's something that I find, with a lot of people, they are very resistant to the thought of completely giving it up. People act like you are taking something away from them, something that is an important part of their life, and you're taking it away forever.

It need not be that way. Just resolve to try a period of abstinence. 30 days. 90 days. Six months. One year. Just try it. You'll live, really. **If you can't do it,** or **you feel as though** you can't do it, that raises all sorts of questions you should be asking yourself, don't you think?

Certain friends gently encouraged me in this direction using wisdom not pressure, and I am eternally grateful to them for that little 'gentle push'. Now I am clear and free from having alcohol in my life, I look at the world of alcohol and what it does to people, with a very clear external view of the effect this psychotropic drug has on people's lives.

To my mind, I think **sugar, alcohol and TV** are the great 'social drugs of our times' and I honestly think life is better with all three gone, but that's just me. Personally, I think hundreds of millions of people are living lives they find confusing, unfulfilling, or spiritually lacking, and they use these three 'social drugs' as crutches, distractions to fill the void. But that's a big old rabbit hole to go down, so I think we'll save that for the next book.

But you may decide to reduce your alcohol consumption to 'moderate' if that works better for you. If you have a healthy relationship with alcohol, great, you should do what works for you, and reducing down to 'moderate' is probably fine. I would say, just try to get it down to a couple of drinks per-week, not a couple of drinks per-day. That's going to see you in a good place.

Benefits of moderate consumption

Many people believe that moderate alcohol consumption is healthier than total abstinence, and this is quite possibly due to the stress-busting benefits of moderate consumption. In turn, reduced stress can mean less heart disease. Of all the studies completed into various health conditions, diseases, longevity and so on, the data gives mixed results. It seems moderate alcohol is associated with slightly better outcomes when it comes to heart disease, than teetotal. However, for most other disease categories, including cancer, dementia, ageing, liver disease and cognitive decline, teetotal seems to be better than moderate consumption. Studies looking at longevity are mixed. Many studies (but not all of them) looking at populations which enjoy extended longevity, show that a glass of red wine over dinner (just the one) every evening is a regular feature of life among many such populations.

The French Paradox

You may have heard that people in France drink more wine than other populations in Europe and yet suffer less heart disease – this is part of what is known as 'The French Paradox' – and this is often cited as evidence that moderate alcohol consumption is good for you. Personally, I think it comes down to how they drink; I think it's more about socialising than drinking. The French consume much of their red wine over a sociable long family lunch or dinner, a gathering with friends, spending time with loved ones. Spending time with people you love and relaxing is a great form of stress relief. Personally, **I think the benefits of moderate alcohol consumption come from stress relief more than anything else.**

Some people say it's the polyphenols in red wine. Maybe it is, but the polyphenols are in the grapes[3], and in spinach, olives, red onions, nuts, cherries, plums and berries too – you don't need to get drunk to enjoy the health benefits of polyphenols in your diet! Sorry for blowing that excuse away!

If a couple of glasses per week, relaxing with friends or family, reduces your stress levels, then that's probably more beneficial for you than harmful, the benefits likely outweigh the harms. But if you use alcohol to drown out a crappy day at work, supping down three or four beers or glasses of wine every night, please don't kid yourself that, "it's good for your heart" because you're drinking too much and that's likely increasing your risk for all manner of other problems.

Drugs

Quite obviously narcotics and recreational drugs are a no-no for a healthy lifestyle. Additionally, you should avoid performance enhancing drugs, steroids, excessive sports stimulants, over-the-counter medications and prescription drugs as much as possible.

Of course, please remember that I am not a doctor, as explained in the 'My Story' chapter earlier, and in the Medical Disclaimer at the back of this book. If your doctor is recommending you take a prescription drug for a specific condition, then you should follow that advice – but you should also talk to your doctor and ask if there might be ways to avoid taking drugs at all. You could ask if healthy dietary and lifestyle options can reduce your need for any drug. Trust me, your doctor will be delighted if you are keen to explore lifestyle and diet modification first, before accepting prescription medications.

---

[3] *Polyphenols produced during red wine ageing.* (Brouillard, R., et al, 1997). See https://www.ncbi.nlm.nih.gov/pubmed/9388306

Remember the 'nine out of ten people just asked for the drugs' story that I shared with you earlier? I have many friends who are doctors and every doctor I know would rather you explored diet and lifestyle options first, before resorting to medications.

Prescription pharmaceuticals certainly play a vital role in our society today, but there are also many cases where such drugs are prescribed too quickly, and patients do not explore all possible alternatives. Many drugs can have side effects or 'knock on' effects, meaning then you need further drugs to deal with those side effects. It can be a cascade, especially in older folks, into something termed polypharmacy.[4]

We encourage you to always look for alternatives to all drugs. *Mother Nature's Diet*, while not a prescription to treat ill health, is a preventive medicine lifestyle designed to try to prevent ill health in the first place. We believe that prevention is better than cure.

Chemicals

Over the last couple of hundred years, we humans have invented around 150,000 chemical compounds[5] that did not exist in Mother Nature's world prior to a thousand years ago. Only a small number of these (less than 10%, but to be honest reports vary and the exact number is not certain) have ever been tested for safety in humans, because the rest are not designed to end up inside us. What do I mean by this? Compounds designed as food additives, for example, are tested for human safety, because they are meant to go in to our food supply. But compounds such as hydraulic fluid, fire retardants, and toilet cleaner, are not tested for human safety (ingestion) because they are not intended for human consumption.

However, experts have discovered traces of between 50% and 75% of all these chemicals do end up inside us...and this is not good news.[6] We simply do not know what effects they are having. Let's face it, the human race has a

---

[4] National Institute for Health and Care Excellence. (2017, January). *Multimorbidity and polypharmacy.* Retrieved from https://www.nice.org.uk/advice/ktt18/chapter/evidence-context

[5] *Scientists categorize Earth as a 'toxic planet'*. (2017, Feb 7). Retrieved from https://m.phys.org/news/2017-02-scientists-categorize-earth-toxic-planet.html

[6] *No Escape: How Fire Retardants Get Into Us.* (2014, Aug 4). Retrieved from https://www.ewg.org/research/flame-retardants-2014/how-fire

blistering track record of messing around with substances that we think are safe, we put them widely into use, and then we figure out they are actually really harmful. Think asbestos, Vioxx, DDT, Thalidomide, BPAs in plastics, and so on.

There are tens of thousands of man-made chemicals out there, untested in humans, yet traces are getting inside us, and we just do not have the science to say whether these compounds are harmful or not. Estimates suggest that at the current rate of testing, it will take us at least another 300 years to get through the chemicals in use today! We can't even be absolutely certain how they end up inside us.

Scientists suggest that:

- We are almost certainly eating traces of pesticides which have been sprayed on our food. Many of these are known to be POPs (Persistent Organic Pollutants) that may be causing serious harm.[7] The long-term effect of multiple pesticide residues accumulating inside us, so far, is not known. Research from 2008, and 2013, is due to be updated in 2019[8]
- It seems likely that we are breathing in fire retardants that are sprayed on our fabrics and soft furnishings in our homes
- Through a process called transdermal absorption,[9] we are absorbing traces of chemicals in cosmetics through our skin (think: they use patches to administer some drugs, such as painkillers, hormone patches, and nicotine patches. By the same mechanism, what about the aluminium or parabens in an under-arm deodorant? Could that be contributing to breast cancer? Many believe so)
- Household and industrial cleaning products end up in our food and on our skin through use and contact
- We are probably breathing in certain bug sprays, air fresheners, body sprays and more

---

[7] Schafer, K.S., & Kegley, S.E. (2002). Persistent toxic chemicals in the US food supply. *BMJ. Journal of Epidemiology & Community Health*, 2002;56:813-817. http://dx.doi.org/10.1136/jech.56.11.813
[8] European Food Safety Authority. (2018, December 5). *Pesticides: new deadline for cumulative risk assessments.* Retrieved from https://www.efsa.europa.eu/en/press/news/181205
[9] See https://en.wikipedia.org/wiki/Transdermal

Somehow, these chemicals are ending up inside us.[10] Many of these chemicals may be what is known as **endocrine disruptors**, that is chemicals that interfere with our regular hormone function. Many may be carcinogenic, that is chemicals that cause cancer. Many may have effects on our brains and neurological function. We just don't know.

With so many questions unanswered, the MND advice is to keep all chemicals in your life to minimum use. Until we have done all the research, which might take the next 300 years, don't use any chemicals unless you really need to. From my own experience, once I cleaned up on the inside, I didn't need to soak my body in deodorant and body spray, because, quite frankly, I didn't smell anymore! I don't need air freshener in my home, just open a window if you need to. I can clean most of my home with Fairy liquid and good old-fashioned 'elbow grease'. I grow my own veg or buy organic. **See, it's actually pretty easy to drop 90% of the chemicals from your home, your food, your skin and your life.** Don't beat yourself up striving for perfection, just do the best you can.

Summary

Core Principle 4 is full of some pretty obvious health advice, like 'quit smoking' and then some rather-less-obvious advice, around alcohol and household chemicals.

What have we learned in this chapter?

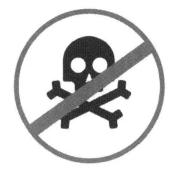

- **Smoking**
- It kills you. Smoking is the #1 preventable cause of death worldwide and here in the UK. 16% of UK deaths in people over 35 years of age are caused by smoking
- It's bloody expensive! Jeez, there are cheaper ways to kill yourself!

---

[10] Rather, I.A., et al. (2017, Nov 17). The Sources of Chemical Contaminants in Food and Their Health Implications. *Frontiers in Pharmacology*, 8: 830. doi: 10.3389/fphar.2017.00830

- The annual cost to society of smoking in England is £14.7bn per annum. The government estimates that for every £1 spent on getting people off the habit, the nation saves £10 in future healthcare costs and health gains
- **Alcohol**
- Contributes to over 200 poor health conditions, including heart disease, several types of cancer, liver disease, depression and more
- Weight gain and obesity
- A quarter of the adult population of England drink too much, above the government recommended safe limit (which, personally, I believe is still set too high)
- "The economic burden of alcohol is estimated between 1.3% and 2.7% of annual GDP." That means the UK loses £739 million per week because of drinking[11]
- Any number of units consumed per week increases your cancer risk
- **You have a choice**
- **One size does not fit all.** If you are good at controlling your relationship with alcohol, then a few drinks per week may be fine for you. If "a few per week" always becomes six per day, maybe you're better off trying abstinence
- The main benefits of moderate consumption are likely stress relief. A few drinks per week may be ideal for a lot of people, but a few drinks per day is too much, for everyone
- **Drugs**
- Don't take drugs for pleasure, that has no place in a healthy lifestyle
- Explore all diet and lifestyle options before resorting to prescription drugs
- Always talk to your doctor first - work with your doctor, he or she would almost certainly love you to find lifestyle changes that help you, rather than taking drugs for many years
- **Chemicals**
- Buy organic
- Don't smother yourself in too many cosmetics and toiletries
- Keep household chemicals to a minimum

---

[11] Mother Nature's Diet blog: *Brexit and booze.* (2017, Nov 7). See https://mothernaturesdiet.me/2017/11/07/brexit-and-booze/

113

You can use this page for your own notes.

Core Principle 5

O xygen is, without question, the most vital nutrient any of us can consume. Every physical, metabolic and physiological process in a human being requires oxygen. OK, now I know, you thought this was 'a diet book' but it's not, it's 'a healthy living book' and that means it's about health, not *just* food. In my opinion, nutrition is really about more than *just* food. Air, water, exercise, sleep, and love are all just as important, or more important, than the food we eat, when it comes to nourishing our bodies. It frustrates me when I see so-called 'diet books' and they are just 300 pages of recipes, and no mention of air, water, sleep, love or exercise. Like those other things don't matter...?

Question: How long can you live without food?
Answer: Months!

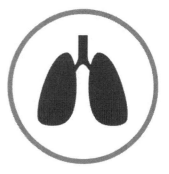

One obese man fasted for over a year (OMG, he did not eat food for a whole year!!), carefully supervised by his doctors, he just drank water and took vitamin and mineral supplements, for just over a year, and he was fine![1]

Q: How long can you live without sleep?
A: It's hard to say as it's virtually impossible (and highly unethical) to test, but from what I can tell, you'd be dead in little over a week, certainly less than a fortnight. And after just a few days, you would be very unwell, very soon.

Q: How long can you live without water?
A: It's about three to four days. See more in the next chapter!

---

[1] Stewart, W.K., & Fleming, L.W. (1973). Features of a successful therapeutic fast of 382 days' duration. BMJ: *Postgraduate Medical Journal*, 49(569), 203-209. From: https://www.ncbi.nlm.nih.gov/pmc/articles/PMC2495396/

Q: How long can you live without love? (Ooh this one will get the science boffins freaking out...am I claiming that love is a 'nutrient'!?!?)
A: Again, it's hard to say, with any degree of scientific certainty, just how important love is for the health of grown adults.

In animal studies, babies will often die in a few days or weeks from something called failure to thrive syndrome (FTTS) if they don't receive maternal attention. FTTS is also well documented in humans, so I think it's fair to say that 'love and human connection' is vital to life. FTTS in humans can be due to many things, not solely lack of parental connection.[2]

In one of the longest running human health studies ever,[3] researchers studied people at around age 50 and then again at age 80, and they concluded that, "quality of relationships" was a more important factor for living to 80 and beyond in good health, than anything else – weight, BMI, cholesterol count, hip-to-waist ratio, blood pressure, etc.[4] I honestly believe that 'love and connection' should be considered a 'nutrient' of sorts - you certainly wouldn't want to live without it.

We must not ignore these factors. Air, water, sleep, love, stress, exercise, are all just as important as the food we do eat, and the food we don't. *Mother Nature's Diet* covers all these dietary and lifestyle factors.

Of course it does! It's a lifestyle, not a fad diet!

Of all these 'nutrients' it's pretty safe to say that air is the most important.

Q: How long can you live without air?
A: Not much more than a few minutes!

Months without food, days without sleep or water, but only minutes without air. I think Mother Nature put them in that order as a clue to show us all how important they are.

---

[2] Johns Hopkins Medicine: *Health Library. Failure to Thrive.* (Undated). Retrieved March 4, 2019, from https://www.hopkinsmedicine.org/healthlibrary/conditions/pediatrics/failure_to_thrive_90,P02297
[3] See the *Harvard Study of Adult Development*, https://www.adultdevelopmentstudy.org/
[4] To learn more, watch the superb TED Talk from Dr Robert Waldinger: *What makes a good life? Lessons from the longest study on happiness.* See https://goo.gl/5Dc9x9

Air (well, oxygen) is the most important nutrient our bodies need. If you don't believe me, try going an hour without it and see how you get on. (Please, don't actually try this!) And yet the irony is, most people pay very little attention to their need for clean fresh air. The majority of people just don't use their lungs enough and just don't get enough fresh clean air every day to truly maximise their health and have abundant natural energy. Core Principles 5 is all about using your lungs more and getting plenty of fresh air every day.

Desk jobs

There are people out there living their entire lives sat down! They wake up in the morning and sit to eat breakfast, and then they sit in the car, and then they sit at their keyboard all morning, and they sit to have lunch, and then they sit back at their keyboard all afternoon, and then they sit in the car and drive home, and then they sit and eat dinner, and then they sit and watch the TV in the evening.

These people are all 'hunched-over' all day, bent over in a position that does not allow their diaphragm a full range of motion, and hence their lungs are never fully expanding and filling completely with air.

Further, they're inside breathing stale air-conditioned air in the office, in the car, and they never get up and move and exert themselves, filling their lungs with fresh air. They're not going out and not getting any exercise. These people aren't breathing properly. This is not just an extreme, there are millions of people in the UK who admit they take no exercise at all, they rarely spend any time outside, and they mostly sit all day every day.

Sadly, this is all too real. This is important stuff. These people are wondering why they're feeling tired all day and nodding off with afternoon slump. They need more oxygen.

Lung health and hunger pangs

Lung health is a big deal, don't downplay this. In the UK, one in five people suffer from a lung or respiratory condition, including asthma, and such conditions are responsible for over one million hospital admissions annually in the UK. **Lung diseases are the third largest cause of death in the UK**, after heart disease and cancer. Lung cancer is the single biggest cancer killer by a large margin. Other big killers include bronchitis and emphysema (collectively known as COPD, chronic obstructive pulmonary disease, a collection of lung conditions), flu and pneumonia.

Upper respiratory tract infections (that is 'persistent coughs, nasty colds and chest infections' in plain English) are among the most common complaints that people present to their GP with.

Additionally, I think a lot of people mistake needing some fresh air as **false hunger pangs**. I think a lot of people are snacking on convenience food (all-too-often poor choices, sugary snacks and drinks) every hour or two of their lives largely because they are either lacking fresh air, or water, or because they are bored, and they are mistaking these feelings for hunger. Often, that short-term feeling of hunger will pass if you grab 60 seconds of fresh air outside, and down a glass of cold water. False hunger pangs pass after about ten minutes, real hunger persists.

Get some vigorous exercise

There are immense health benefits to be gained from making your lungs work maximally on a regular basis. We will look at exercise in much more detail in Core Principle 9, but for now just understand that there is a time and place in life for gentle exercise, and a time and place for vigorous exercise.

Vigorous can mean different things to different people – again, **one size does not fit all.** The idea is to do something that gets your heart thumping and your lungs working at full capacity, so that means exercise at 'high intensity' whatever that means to you. To one person, that's a brisk walk, to another person that's a maximum-effort sprint.

Pushing your lungs to work hard from time to time will help maintain your lung function and lung capacity as you age. Personally, I am a big believer in the idea of 'use it or lose it' and I think we can apply that to many things in life, such as fitness, strength, flexibility, brain power, our sex lives and more. One thing is lung function. We need to get our lungs working at maximum capacity once a week to ensure we maintain lung function as we age. That means regular aerobic exercise is a must. Running, swimming, cycling, rowing or just brisk, hilly walking, it doesn't matter what, but you need to get out at least once or twice per week and get puffing and panting. In many ways, your life depends on it!!

If jogging, swimming and cycling don't appeal to you, join a sports club and play a sport you enjoy, like tennis, hockey, netball or football. If it makes you run around for an hour once or twice per week, that's perfect.

Take a break

If you have an office job and you want to have more energy, get out every day, go for a walk, go out at lunch time, go take a ten- or twenty-minute stroll, get some air into your body, energise yourself. There are so many simple ways you can get more movement into your working day and hence more oxygen into your body. Use a car park that's further away from the office, and walk the extra ten minutes in to work every morning. Get a dog, go out for an early morning walk every day. If you've got a meeting two floors up, don't take the lift, run up the stairs. Take your boxed salad for lunch and go eat it in the park. Make it happen!

Beauty is only skin deep

We all want to resist the signs of ageing the best we can. That includes wanting to have good, soft, blemish and wrinkle free skin. There are many factors involved in having good skin, one of them is oxygen. Your skin does not suck up oxygen from the outside, you have to feed it oxygen from the inside – via your blood. Healthy blood transports oxygen around the body, feeding it to all your muscles and organs, including your skin. Using your lungs, getting plenty of fresh air, staying active, and getting some exercise a few times per week all helps to maintain youthful good skin.

Summary

Core Principle 5: Breathe! Use your lungs fully, get plenty of fresh air, every day. If you want to live a long and healthy life, you need to look after your lungs. Remember, every single process in the human body needs oxygen. Oxygen is about as vital as it gets, you're dead in just a few minutes without it.

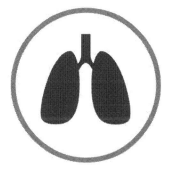

- Nutrition is about more than just food

- Any 'diet program' that only talks about food is far from complete. Air, water, sleep, exercise, love and sunlight are all important factors in any healthy lifestyle
- Breathe deeply, move your diaphragm, let your tummy out, fill your lungs and move your body
- Lack of oxygen can be a root cause behind lethargy, tiredness, afternoon slump and false hunger pangs
- Get outside, get fresh air and sunshine every day, exert yourself with a brisk walk and breathe deeply
- Lung health is important, use it or lose it, use your lungs
- Exercise a few times per week at low to moderate intensity to keep maximum amounts of oxygen moving around your body every day
- Try to exercise at maximal effort at least once per week. Cycle up a big hill, sprint around your local park or do a HiiT workout at the gym
- Country air is much cleaner than city air, so get out and enjoy the countryside whenever you can. If you live in a city – go to the park!
- Oxygen is good for your skin too, so exercise and fresh air help to keep you looking youthful

There are numerous other aspects of breathing that we could look into in this chapter, such as deep breathing techniques, breathing exercises for stress relief, diaphragmatic breathing, yoga breathing techniques, breathing exercises for COPD, breathing to increase lung capacity, power breathing, breathing techniques in running and endurance sports, meditative breathing, mindful breathing - but other people have already written books on all those topics, so if these are areas that you feel you want to look into closer, then I would encourage you to go do further research on your own.

In this book, I am trying to keep things simple, as much as possible, to help you to understand these basic concepts of healthy living, and I am trying to avoid deep diving into every topic in infinite detail. We've looked at air, now let's move on to water.

Core Principle 6

D rinking lots of clean water is an essential element of a healthy lifestyle. Think about it, as we saw in the last chapter, you can live for several months without food, but *you will die after just three to four days without any water.* Water is seriously important stuff, yet the majority of 'diet books' rarely give it a mention. Roughly 60% to 65% of a human body is made up of water,[1] so don't underestimate your need to hydrate well every day.

Most of your brain is made of water, your skin has high water content and half of your blood is water. Water is a major component of all human body organs, and without water intake, *you will go from perfectly healthy to dead in a little over three days.* Among other things, water regulates body temperature, aids digestion, mineral absorption and bowel function, helps to lubricate joints, aids cell regeneration and helps your body to manufacture vital hormones.

Water is vital to life, and vital to feeling good and functioning well. The **acute symptoms** of **dehydration** include headaches, irregular sleep, tiredness, loss of strength and energy, weariness, constipation, dry flaky skin and scalp, mental confusion, depression, muscle cramps, sunken eyes, lethargy, fever, dizziness, loss of orientation, vomiting, low blood pressure, irregular heartbeat, palpitations, loss of consciousness, multiple organ failures and death. It is quite incredible how fast dehydration can wipe you out. You can literally go from 100% healthy, through this whole list to death all in under four days, and then that's it, game over.

We must not under estimate the importance of good hydration if you want abundant healthy living! If *mild dehydration* can cause headaches,

---

[1] U.S. Geological Survey website. *The water in you.* Read more at https://water.usgs.gov/edu/propertyyou.html

tiredness, lethargy, weariness, loss of strength, constipation and depression, it seems to me that *good hydration* well may be the 'cure' to many *mild cases of these conditions*. I meet people all the time who complain of such symptoms – headaches, weariness, lethargy, constipation and mild depression. I ask them how much water they drink most days and the answer is almost always very little or none!

It's important to ensure you drink at least two litres of water every day. That number is not an exact science...a big person may need more; a small person may need less. You will likely need more if you are exercising hard or if it is hot weather and you are sweating a lot, and some days you may get away with less. Just remember that good hydration is an essential cornerstone of a healthy lifestyle.

False hunger and weight loss

Often times, when our body wants water, we mistake the feeling of thirst for hunger. I see my kids doing this all the time, at the weekend, they haven't had a drink of water for at least a couple of hours, maybe several hours, and suddenly they are cruising the kitchen for snacks, asking "when's lunch" and thinking they are hungry. In fact, a glass of water does the trick and that hunger passes, in minutes it's gone.

Kids can get away with that mistake, but many overweight older adults can't. Habitually snacking is many people's downfall when it comes to eating the wrong foods and slowly gaining the pounds over a long period of time. Remember that often when people think they are hungry, really, they are just slightly dehydrated, they just need a drink of water. As we noted in the previous chapter, lack of fresh air, and a lack of fresh water, can lead to false hunger pangs. In our modern world, carbohydrate-based snacks like crisps, sweets, cakes and biscuits, are never far away, and all too often people are snacking between meals, adding hundreds of calories per day to their diet, when what they really need is a five-minute movement break, a few lung-fulls of fresh air, and a glass of water.

Sexy soft skin

Your skin is around 65% to 70% water by weight, so good hydration is a key element to keeping your skin nourished, soft and supple. Can you see, again and again, how we keep coming back to these same points? Want to resist the signs of ageing, want to keep your skin soft? Well the 'secrets' are all here – a high nutrient diet, good proteins, vitamins and minerals, not smoking, plenty of oxygen, fresh air and time outside, and good hydration. As you read the rest of this book, we'll add sleep, responsible sun exposure and regular daily exercise to that list. You see, **resisting the signs of ageing – you have a choice**. You have *more control* over this than you might have previously thought. It's a key theme of this book, I shall keep repeating it!

Whenever I meet one of those women who has beautiful glowing soft skin and looks a decade younger than she is, I'll get health habits into the conversation and I always find that good hydration is a cornerstone. I don't think I ever hear, "Oh my secret is this magic night cream I put on, it's about 50 quid for this tiny pot but it's gold…" Nope. What I hear is – good hydration and good sleep, and no smoking and boozing! They drink water and not alcohol, that's one of the big secrets to youthful good skin!

Can you drink too much?

You may have read bizarre stories in the press of people dying from drinking too much water. Or you may read articles warning you to watch out for crazy people on the Internet who are not qualified doctors (uh oh, people like me!!!) telling everyone to drink lots of water every day, when in fact there is no science to back this up.

Is any of that true? Well, you certainly can drink too much, if you're not very active. If you have too much, you're diluting some of your body's store of certain minerals, such as sodium, and then this can be a problem. But in reality, your body has clever systems to maintain the balance between water and sodium (called homeostasis) and so if you have too much of one or the other, your body adjusts to help restore the correct balance.

If you are sensible, and drink around 1.5 litres to 2.5 litres per day, then more if you are very active, sweating a lot or in very warm weather, then everything should balance out OK.

Indeed, some people have died of drinking too much water, but it's not actually quite as clear-cut as that. When you drink too much water, you don't die because your body can't handle the water, you die because you dilute your sodium so much that you develop a condition called hyponatremia, and this can quite quickly lead to heart failure.

As mentioned above, your body works very hard all day long to keep sodium and water in balance in the body (homeostasis). If you do something drastic that causes you to lose a lot of water, like running an ultramarathon in warm sunny weather, and then you go to replace *only* the water very quickly, by guzzling lots, **without** also replacing lost sodium (and other minerals called electrolytes) at the same time, then what sodium you do have is massively diluted, and that's when you can wind up in big trouble. It's quite rare, but it can happen, and it can be fatal.

If you do a lot of exercise and sweat profusely, get in the habit of putting the electrolytes back in with the water (you can buy electrolyte drinks or supplements) and everything will stay in balance and you'll be fine. Realistically, if you're the kind of person out there running ultramarathons in hot weather, you likely know that already - well, I hope so!!

Water, water everywhere, nor any drop to drink

Water is one of the most important essential nutrients we need in any healthy diet. I suggest the average person drinks approximately two litres per day, and then add more to replace sweat lost due to strenuous exercise and hot weather. Two litres equates to around eight regular-sized kitchen 'highball' glasses per day.

> **"Mild dehydration can cause headaches, tiredness, lethargy, weariness, loss of strength, constipation and depression. It seems to me that good hydration well may be the cure to many mild cases of these conditions."**
>
> Something to think about there! Stay well hydrated!

Summary

- Drink water for energy and vigour – even mild dehydration causes lethargy and fatigue
- Water helps you to maintain lovely soft, youthful, supple skin
- You need water for good bowel function – slight dehydration is a classic cause of constipation

- Drink plenty of water for good brain function. Your brain is mostly made of fat and water, and cholesterol, interestingly, so drink water for good brain function – that includes treating acute cases of depression
- Headaches are a classic first sign of mild dehydration, so if you are prone, drink up!
- Drink a glass of water to stave off false hunger pangs
- Drinking more water can help treat some dry or flaky skin conditions
- Drink water in combination with a high-nutrient diet, to ensure you are replacing your electrolytes (minerals) along with water lost during exercise

You can use this page for your own notes.

Core Principle 7

Just eat real food. Through Core Principle 1 to 4 we took all the things out of our diet that are not benefitting us. We took out most of the bulky starchy foods, we cut the refined sugar, the processed foods that encourage over-eating, and we pulled away from the smoking and drinking.

Now we've cleared that unhealthy stuff off your plate, it's time to put the good stuff back in. In very simple terms, we only really want to eat **real food**, that's basically plants and animals.

> "If you can imagine it in your mind's eye, swimming, flying, running, crawling, hanging on a tree, sprouting up out of the ground on a bush or a root, then broadly speaking, that's real food."

If you really think about what food Mother Nature put on this earth for us humans to eat, if you think about what was naturally available as food for humans before we built shops and roads, boats and planes, tractors and refrigerated warehouses, it all comes down to **plants and animals**. We ate plants and animals, and we drank **water**.

Anatomically modern man, Homo Sapiens, has lived on Earth for around 185,000 years. In broad terms, for about 184,700 of those years we ate plants and animals and drank water. There were no fridge-freezers, no sugar-coated hoop-shaped multi-coloured breakfast cereals, no fizzy drinks, no oven pizzas and no convenience stores selling bags of crisps and chocolate bars.

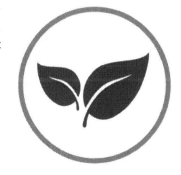

You might have read the last paragraph and thought this is all sounding like a spin on the Paleo diet or something similar. Paleo is great, on my own personal health journey to creating MND, I 'came through Paleo' and I still follow the work of the original experts in this area, such as Mark Sisson, Robb Wolf and Loren Cordain, and I highly recommend those guys and their books. However, while thinking about our ancestors and our origins, it is also important to remember that almost nothing on Earth in the 21st century is still as it was in the Paleolithic era, not 50,000 years ago, 200,000 years ago, or a million years ago.

Almost all plants today have been changed by farming through hundreds of years of selective breeding. Topsoil composition has changed, as has air to some degree (we have pollution now) and fresh water and sea water. Animals have been bred to be smaller, or larger, fatter, or leaner, more muscular or faster growing. Foods are now grown using chemical inputs including pesticides, hormone supplements and artificial fertilisers. We have GMOs. We have electric lighting and different sleep patterns. We have sedentary jobs and different activity patterns. Almost everything is different. Trying to emulate a previous time in evolutionary history is almost impossible, but we can look back at those previous times and learn.

The reality is that very few of the things we can buy in our shops as food today are the same as they were back tens of thousands of years ago.

"In my opinion, the best thing we can do to emulate the more natural diet of our ancient ancestors is to 'eat plants and animals' and do our best to avoid processed foods. It's all in the 12 Core Principles."

In my opinion, the best thing we can do to emulate the more natural diet of our ancient ancestors is to 'eat plants and animals' and do our best to avoid processed foods – as laid out in Core Principles 1, 2 and 3 of *Mother Nature's Diet*. Once we take out all that processed stuff, Core Principle 7 and 8 are all about putting the good stuff in instead, by eating fresh, natural, whole foods.

Plants (we're talking vegetables, and some fruits, nuts and seeds)

There are many great reasons to eat lots of vegetables and fruits in your daily diet, especially vegetables.

- Eating lots of veggies and fruits means lots of micronutrients – vitamins and minerals – which are good for you in a great many ways, as we have discussed
- Eating a lot of veggies displaces most of the processed starchy 'beige bloat food' from your dinner plate, and adds beneficial **fibre** to your diet. High fibre content is one of the main reasons the World Health Organisation promote the 5-a-day idea, because fibre in your diet helps combat colorectal cancers
- Replacing the grains and starchy carbs in your meals for more vegetables exchanges those calories we talked about in Core Principle 1, for more nutritious high-fibre foods

Less calories, more nutrients. Do you remember? That's one of our main goals...that's a big reason why we want to cut a lot of the cereals, bread and pasta, and eat more vegetables instead.

One of the core goals of the MND lifestyle is to consume a very nutrient-dense diet. We want well-above-normal levels of vitamins and minerals, and we really don't want to waste our time, money, or our 'digestive energy' eating low-nutrient-density foods, that offer calories but little in the way of vitamins and minerals. Micronutrients are important for powering all our bodily functions, resisting ill health and helping us to have lots of energy, so we want to eat as many nutrient-rich foods as we can.

Lots of vegetables are great, and let's not forget fruits too. Our healthy lifestyle should include a couple of portions of fruit every day, again because fruit offers lots of beneficial micronutrients and some additional dietary fibre. Citrus fruits, berries (tend to be seasonal) and bananas all offer useful nutrients, and many find apples, pears or similar offer just the right amount of fibre to maintain healthy bowel function. Personally, I find an apple a day provides ideal fibre for optimal regular bowel function, and one piece of citrus fruit per day offers a great vitamin C top up. I also grow berries at home, so eat lots of colourful berries in the summer months.

Misconceptions about veggies

While it might be tempting to think that vegetables are some kind of wonder foods, that maybe we should all become vegetarians for a long and healthy life, we also need to eat animal foods, as they too offer many benefits, and in fact animal foods are, in many respects, more beneficial and nutrient dense than plant foods.

There are some persistent myths around the health benefits of vegetarianism and the idea that all plants are good for us, and that we only need to eat plants and we can abandon animal foods. Check out my 'Myth Busting' series on the *Mother Nature's Diet* blog[1] to get the straight facts on these issues. The truth is that we need to eat animal foods too; without question, animal foods are the most nutrient-dense foods on the planet.

Animals (meat, fish and eggs)

Animal foods contain many vital nutrients that we need. Meat and fish will give you the best proteins available, called 'complete proteins' and these really are the building blocks of all life. You may have heard that plant foods (vegetables) contain protein too, and that's true, they do, but they are not complete proteins, they are what's known as 'incomplete proteins' and as such – without going in to too much detail – they are inferior proteins to that which you will get from eggs, meat and fish.

Animal foods also contain some of the best essential fats. We ideally want to get lots of good fats in our diet, and cut down on the bad fats. There is more on fats coming up in the next chapter, but for now let's understand that oily fish, free range eggs, grass-fed meats, grass-fed butter and cream, and good-quality fattier meats (like chicken thigh instead of breast, and roast pork) are also great sources of healthy beneficial, nutritious fats.

Animal foods are also by far the most nutrient-dense foods on the planet. By far. If I have convinced you in this book so far that you want a nutrient-dense diet, then consuming animal foods is a key element of that diet.

---

[1] See the *Mother Nature's Diet* blog here for more reading:
https://mothernaturesdiet.me/2016/04/27/myth-busting-part-3/

Some of the key nutritional benefits of animal foods include:

- Vitamin A is much more bioavailable from meat than from non-animal sources, by a factor of 1000% or more
- Some of the best sources of B group vitamins (B1, B2, B3 and B6) are animal foods such as liver, fish, eggs and pork
- Vitamin B12 is mostly only found in animal foods. Some B12 can be found in vegetables, but not in a form that is bio-available to the human digestive system
- Vitamin D is not found in plants at all, it is only found in animal foods. (Alternatively, your body can use sunlight to convert cholesterol into vitamin D)
- Iron from animal sources is far more bioavailable than from plant sources, it's a different form of iron completely. Your body really wants haem iron, which comes from animal foods
- EPA and DHA (fatty acids, these are health-promoting omega-3 fatty acids) are only found in animal foods, mostly in oily fish and fish oils. These fatty acids are essential for brain and nervous system function, and omega-3 fatty acids have been shown in many studies to promote heart health

All these nutrients are important and their bioavailability from animal sources is far better than from plant sources. Over a period of years, a vegetarian diet, and particularly a vegan diet, *can potentially* lead to a number of nutritional deficiencies, such as vitamin B6 and B12, iron, and certain important fatty acids. Eating animal products such as oily fish, eggs and organ meats (such as kidneys and liver), ensures we correct these imbalances. Alternatively, most vegans will source these nutrients from synthetic supplements, particularly B12.

Plants and animals

As you can now see, a balanced, healthy, optimally-nutritious diet should ideally be made up of foods coming from both plants and animals, as both offer beneficial nutrients. *Mother Nature's Diet* recommends that around half of your calories should be coming from meat, fish and eggs, and the other half of your calories from vegetables, fruits, nuts and seeds. That's the MND way.

Do you remember we looked at 'The Eatwell Plate' back in the chapter on micronutrients? You may recall it looks like this.

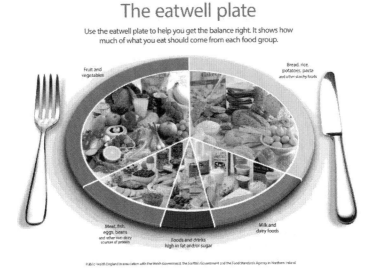

Well, now we have our own *Mother Nature's Diet* version.

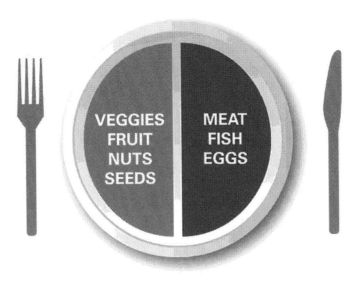

We want to get around half of our total calories from plants, and the other half of our calories from animals. However, the animal foods tend to be much more calorie dense than plant foods, because they contain more fats, which are more calorie-dense than proteins or carbohydrates. Therefore, in reality, what you are actually going to see on your plate, is around one third of your food will be meat, or fish, or eggs, and then the other two thirds of your plate will be filled with vegetables or a salad.

I often say that a "palm sized" piece of meat is adequate for an average meal. That might be a chicken breast or thigh, or a pork or lamb chop, something like that. Then fill the rest of your plate with vegetables, or a big fresh salad. Of course, we know that one size does not fit all, so there may be some variation if you are an athlete or if you are training for some special event, or maybe you just fancy something different, but as a general guideline, and if a healthy diet and weight loss are your goals, this should work well for most people.

Putting your meals together this way, your MND food plate is going to look pretty much like this. Really, that's all pretty simple, isn't it?

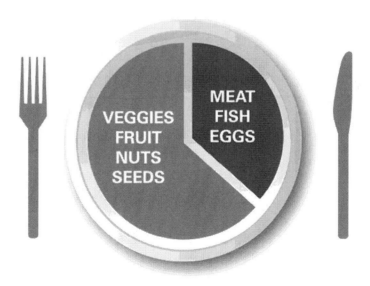

Finally, **fresh fruits and nuts** may be used as snacks, for the main part. What you are going to end up with might look something like this last image.

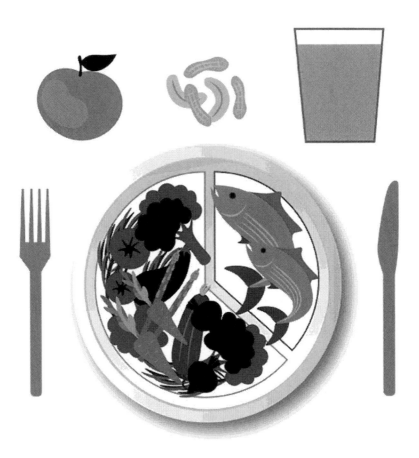

A serving of fish, lots of fresh vegetables, boiled, steamed, roasted or stir-fried, and you're all set. An apple for a morning snack, a few nuts for an afternoon or evening snack *if required*, and water to drink throughout the day, and hot teas and coffees if you like. Easy, tasty, nutritious.

A balanced healthy diet

Ideally, you should look to create variety and balance in your diet; try to get some of your protein from meat, some from fish, some from eggs. Don't get stuck eating only one thing. I meet some people who eat lean white chicken breast every day and never any other meat. They have been scared away from animal fats over the last 40 years because of the anti-fat message from the diet industry, which is wrong in my opinion. (Don't worry, we'll make sense of fats in the next chapter.)

That's a mistake, you should not avoid animal fats, because you need the vital nutrients in those good fats to help your body absorb other nutrients. For example, your body uses vitamin A to synthesise and assimilate proteins. If you only eat lean meats, and avoid fatty meats (such as fish, fish oils, liver, chicken thighs, pork, beef and eggs) then you might be slowly depleting your body of vitamin A, and you may not be absorbing and assimilating the protein you eat properly. Equally don't *only* eat tinned tuna; instead eat a variety of fish. Don't *only* eat broccoli; eat lots of different greens. Don't *only* eat carrots; opt for lots of coloured veggies. Don't get stuck on just one thing.

Aim to eat a wide variety of vegetables, look for all the different colours – greens, reds, yellows, etc., as colour often indicates a variety of different available micronutrients.

Aim to eat a variety of fish, especially oily fish (salmon, herring, mackerel, pilchards/sardines), meats of all sorts, including organ meats such as liver and kidneys, and free-range eggs. Don't deny children foods with good fats in them. We have seen the diet industry and many health experts push an agenda of 'fat is bad' and 'cholesterol is bad' for the last 40 or 50 years, yet many scientists[2] and doctors[3] argue that there is not one scrap of evidence that total dietary cholesterol causes any harm at all to human health.[4]

Cholesterol is an essential component of all cells in all animals. Cholesterol forms an essential element of all cell membranes in your body, it holds cells together and without any you would be dead. In terms of your ability to live and survive, it's as important as air, water, blood and glucose for the brain – it's absolutely essential. It is so important, that all animals can produce their own cholesterol; so if there is not enough coming in your diet, your body will make more for itself.

Ask yourself this question: Cholesterol is present in every single cell in the human body, and it is so important that if you don't eat enough of it in your diet, then your body will make more so that you have enough. Do you really think Mother Nature would evolve this substance that is so essential to life, that you make it inside, and yet it gives you heart disease and kills you?

To me, that doesn't make any sense at all. Ummm, another thing to ponder. [More on the topic of cholesterol in the FAQs at the end of this book.] Me, I don't buy it. Personally, I think the whole cholesterol debate is wide open and misguided. I think the research is flawed and we'll see 'the official story' change in the coming decades.

Loading up your nutrient dense diet

You want your diet high in nutrient dense foods. Remember, the plague of the modern Western world is that too many people are **over-fed, but under-nourished.** Therefore, our goal in general, as a population, is to eat fewer calories but more nutrients.

- You want to get **oily fish** on your plate, perhaps three, four, or five times per week

---

[2] Harcombe, Z. (2017). Dietary fat guidelines have no evidence base: where next for public health nutritional advice? *British Journal of Sports Medicine*, 51, 769-774. http://dx.doi.org/10.1136/bjsports-2016-096734
[3] See The International Network of Cholesterol Skeptics: http://www.thincs.org/members.php
[4] *Greater Cholesterol lowering increases the risk of death*. (2016, April 13). Retrieved from https://drmalcolmkendrick.org/2016/04/13/greater-cholesterol-lowering-increases-the-risk-of-death/

- You should look to include some **grass-fed** meat in your diet a couple of times per week
- Try to ensure you get some **free-range** eggs a few times per week
- It would be extremely beneficial to eat some **organ meat** such as liver or kidney at least once per week
- Eat lots of **fresh vegetables every day**, look to eat **all the colours**, greens, reds, yellows, oranges and more
- Include some **citrus fruit** several times per week
- Include good plant fats too, such as **olives,** olive oil, **nuts and seeds** (like flax seeds) and avocado, these are all excellent healthy plant fats

Personally, I will eat a serving of oily fish such as mackerel or sardines, with around six to eight servings of green vegetables (that's a lot of veg!) for breakfast several times per week (alternating eggs or fish). I usually get up at 6am, have a glass of water and walk my dog, then do an hour's work with a coffee, then have breakfast a couple of hours after getting up. I work from home most of the time so I have that flexibility with my schedule.

But I appreciate that might sound a bit 'hard core' to you if you are used to having cereal and toast or something like that! It's OK, I get it...it's not like I went in *one day* from my bowl of sugar-coated cereal and peanut butter on toast, straight to the mackerel and kale for breakfast! No, I transitioned over several years, as explained earlier, while I was learning about health and nutrition. Remember, as I keep saying, it's all about **progress, not perfection**.

Just start.

With my super nutritious breakfast packed in, my lunch is likely to be a salad, perhaps with some ham, or chicken, or hard-boiled eggs, or maybe a little feta cheese made from goat's milk. If I need snacks during the day then I'll have an apple and maybe a grapefruit or an orange, and I may nibble some nuts, like almonds or walnuts, but not too many. Then finally dinner is likely to be a little palm sized piece of meat or fish with lots of vegetables or a big salad.

I will drink three or four cups of black decaf coffee in the morning, lots of water all day, and probably a couple of herbal teas in the afternoon. How easy does that sound? That's it, a regular day. Plants and animals. Big focus on nutrients. It's just not that hard to do.

Try to be a lover of liver

If you can, learn to love liver. I know that's another tough call for a lot of people. Maybe like me you have flashbacks to the plate load of rubbery stuff swimming in gravy that my mum used to force-feed me once a month, despite my complaints and protestations. Well, actually, if we learn how to cook liver and kidneys properly, they can be delicious. Organ meats are literally, hands-down, the most nutritious foods on the planet. Liver wins, bar none, it's jam-packed with nutrients. If you can get some liver into your diet, even if it's just once per month, your body sure will thank you for it. Nutritionally speaking, organ meats are fantastic value-for-money.

Liver pâté is pretty easy to make yourself at home if you have a blender, just check on Google for a recipe and instructions. Look for liver on the menu in restaurants when you dine out. It's made a bit of a resurgence in recent years and some restaurants serve fantastic tasty liver dishes. Otherwise, at home, I'll sometimes add liver to a curry or a chilli-con-carne, chop some up and mix it in and lose it in the flavours, and hope the kids don't notice!

Summary of Core Principle 7

Plants and animals!! That's it, plants and animals are the only 'real food' on planet Earth, everything else is somehow a processed, adulterated or man-made form of 'edible food products' but the truth remains that everything comes from plants and animals in the first place.

Cut out most of the processed crap and just eat plants and animals!

- Meat and poultry
- Organ meats
- Fish, shell fish and all seafood
- Vegetables
- Fruits
- Nuts and seeds
- Water

Focus your efforts on ensuring that **at least 90% of your diet** is made up of these wonderful nourishing, fresh whole foods, and you'll be ticking all the right boxes.

Remember the key points here:

- We don't want to spend our money on packaging and ad campaigns, we want to spend our precious shopping budget on real food, nutrition
- Fresh whole foods are far more nutrient-dense than processed foods
- The most nutrient-dense foods on Earth are animal foods
- All the different coloured vegetables provide lots of valuable micronutrients, plus vegetables give us insoluble fibre (good for your gut bacteria, the beneficial ones) and beneficial starches (in small amounts)
- Fruits give us vitamins and soluble fibre (helps keep you regular!)
- Nuts and seeds for good fats
- Organic, grass-fed dairy as a condiment
- A balanced diet includes fish, meat, organ meats and free-range eggs every week, and fresh fruits and vegetables every day
- Keep things simple: approximately one third of your plate contains a protein source such as meat, fish or eggs, then the other two thirds of the plate are filled with vegetables or salad

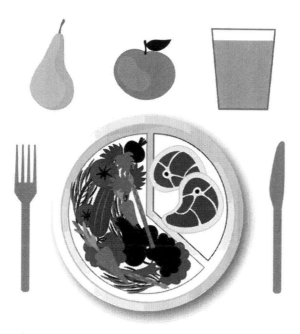

You can use this page for your own notes.

Sidebar: The Facts on Fats

BUSTING THE BULL***T!

There are so many frustrating myths permeating in the weight loss, health and fitness world. If you read my story you know this is something that frustrated the heck out of me for a very long time. The conflicting advice, conflicting research and conflicting expert opinions is enough to drive anyone crazy! No wonder the public are so confused and fed up by all this nonsense.

Eating fat won't make you fat

Let's straighten out a few facts about dietary fats. You shouldn't be afraid of eating fat. **If it's 'good fat'** or 'natural fat' then it's good for you. Ah how the devil is in the detail!

This, then, begs the question: **what is good fat**, or 'natural' fat? Well, oily fish are very fatty, but it's good fat, it's an important part of the fish, and it's very healthy for us, so that's a natural good fat – the fat is part of the fish, and fish is one of the most abundant food sources on Earth. 71% of the planet is covered with water, and our ancient ancestors ate seafood for tens of thousands of years, so fish are a very 'natural' food source for us, and fish is an important source of natural healthy fat that we should include in our balanced healthy diet.

What about the fat in, say, beef? Now let's see how this same 'natural' fat argument stacks up for a cow. Of course, there is fat on a cow – I mean, I bet you have never seen a cow with a rippling 6-pack, right? The two things to think about are, 1) how much fat is on the cow, and 2) what kind of fat is it?

Wild ruminants (a cow is a ruminant) like caribou, reindeer and wildebeest, typically have quite low levels of bodyfat (they are pretty 'ripped' in the ruminant world!) because they live an active life, on the move, always searching for food, always moving away from predators, and in many cases undergoing an annual migration between winter lands and summer lands.

Therefore, wild ruminants are always moving and always competing for food – in today's modern diet-world terminology they 'eat less, and move more' all the time, and as a result, these wild animals are pretty lean.

By comparison, many farmed ruminants (we are mostly talking about cows here) stand around in a barn for most of their time, eating all day, and not expending much energy to compete for their food. They are also fed grains, corn, soybeans and other staples that help to 'fatten them up' because this is the goal for most farmers, to grow their livestock big and heavy, as quickly as possible, ready to sell (by the pound) at market. In modern-day diet parlance, these ruminants 'eat more than they need and don't move very much'. The net result is obese cows.

What does this mean for your beef? Well it means that the beef we buy in our supermarkets, is likely to be far fattier than the meat we would get from wild animals. Simply, there is likely to be more fat on a farmed animal than on a wild animal.

I said our second consideration should be the *kind of fat* we get from beef. Again, if the animal is a wild animal, it's diet will have been composed pretty much entirely of grass and meadow flowers and weeds, and probably some leaves. The food the animal eats, determines the mineral content and the fatty acid composition of its meat – what that means is, a grass-fed cow will have meat that is high in omega-3 fatty acids. You have probably heard that omega-3 fatty acids are good for you, for your brain function, your joints, your heart and more.

By contrast, if our farmed cow has spent much of its life in a shed, eating corn, soybeans and other grains, then its meat will contain more omega-6 fatty acids, these are the type of fatty acids we want less of in our diet.

Therefore, to answer the question – is beef fat good or bad? Is it a 'healthy natural fat' or not, then the answer comes down to this:

If the cow was free ranged and grass fed, then the fat in the beef should be a healthy natural fat, but if the cow spent its entire life in a barn eating grains, corn and soybeans, then the beef is likely to be higher in fat than it should be, and the fat will not be a healthy natural fat.

You can see, the answer to whether or not eating meat, such as beef, is good for you or not, is nuanced. It might be fair to say...

There's beef, and then there's beef.

I don't know if you have spotted it yet, but there is something of a pattern forming here.

- On Page 52 we saw: There's bread, and then there's bread
- And then on Page 102: There's milk, and there's milk
- Now here we see: There's beef, and then there's beef

Maybe you can see now, this is all a part of the reason why diet advice has become so confusing over the years. Some days you read a newspaper article claiming "Eating red meat gives you colon cancer" or "Bread makes you fat" or "Cow's milk promotes breast cancer" or "Saturated fat causes heart disease" or some similar horror story.

The very next week we read that there is no link between red meat and colon cancer; that whole grain bread is 'the staff of life' and has been a healthy diet staple for thousands of years; that diary food is important for women and helps prevent osteoporosis; and that saturated fat is health promoting and good for us.

It's no wonder folks get so confused and frustrated - I did! The reality is nuanced. There is no one size fits all. We (people) are all different, and the food products are all different. There's bread, and then there's bread. There's milk, and then there's milk. Same for the beef. The pork. Cheese. Yoghurt. Fruit. The list goes on and on. Can you see?

Let's circle back to the beef. How the heck does anyone make sense of all this in an average British supermarket? **The short answer is – buy organic.** There are top-of-the-range options we can all aspire to, such as meat approved by the PFLA, the Pasture-Fed Livestock Association, or meat sold as Soil Association Organic, or we can seek out local farm shops selling 100% grass-fed or 100% pasture-raised meat. But in reality, I realise that for many people, these options simply will not be available. So, if you just want to make the best choice possible, buy organic.

For British supermarkets like Sainsbury's and Tesco to sell beef labelled organic, the cows have to be free ranged (this information is correct at time of writing), which means they spend most of their lives outside mainly eating grass. Those cows will likely have eaten some grains too, but it's about doing the best we can.

For most of us, realistically, this is our best bet. (See that, an example of 'progress, not perfection'.) When we buy organic beef, we are eating 'good fats' but when we buy the regular cheaper stuff, then we are likely buying beef that is higher in fat, and it's not the good fat.

Keeping things simple

My goal in these pages is not to provide an exhaustive analysis of this subject and cover everything there is to know about dietary fat. That's a vast topic that could (and does) fill entire books on its own.[1] We just need to understand that some fats are broadly natural and have been in our diet for eons, while other fats are not-so-natural, they are products of the industrialisation of agriculture, and we're better off keeping those fats to a minimum in our diet.

Can you now see how *Mother Nature's Diet* makes sense of our health and our food, by connecting human health, with good standards in farming, with animal welfare, and with what's best for the environment? I called it *Mother Nature's Diet* because so often, looking to Mother Nature for the natural way things should be done, provides us with the answers we are looking for, for our best health and longevity. 'Eat plants and animals' is a great example of taking all that complexity, and making it simple.

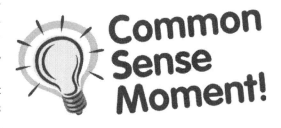

Here at MND, we don't see all these areas as separate issues, we see it all as one big picture. And it **all has one set of answers**. What's right for your health, is also best for animal welfare, best for the farmers, and best for the environment. ***Joined up thinking.*** *It's how it should be.*

---

[1] If you're interested, try *The Big Fat Surprise*, an excellent book by Nina Teicholz. 2015. See https://www.amazon.co.uk/Big-Fat-Surprise-butter-healthy/dp/192522810X/

Sure, that organic labelled food is going to cost you a few quid more per week. But what you spend extra on organic food, you'll save on drinking less alcohol and buying fewer take-aways. It's about making better choices. It's about doing the right thing.

Vegetable oils and trans fats

The worst kind of fats around, the ones we really want to avoid, are trans fats. These are not such a big deal these days as they were a decade or two ago, as public awareness and consumer action have successfully pushed the food companies to remove a lot of the trans fats from our food.

Trans fats do occur naturally at low levels in some foods, mostly in animal foods, but in pretty small quantities. Where trans fats started to appear in large amounts was in processed foods that used hydrogenated vegetable and seed oils. Pastries, junk food and particularly margarine and shortening, these foods were key places where trans fats came into our diet. Trans fats are associated with increased rates of heart disease[2] and some studies have linked trans fats with increased risks of colon cancer and breast cancer.[3]

Most of the trans fats have now been removed from these foods, and of course we avoid those foods anyway living the MND way (Core Principle 3). Avoid margarines and vegetable seed oils, and keep away from processed foods, and that should keep your trans fats consumption very low.

Palm oil

Frustratingly, one of the ways food manufacturers cut those trans fats out, was to replace them with palm oil! Now palm oil has become the most widely cultivated vegetable oil on Earth, and it's "the new fat that everyone loves to hate" because of its cost to the environment. Growing oil palms is a major

---

[2] Iqbal, M.P. (2014). Trans fatty acids – A risk factor for cardiovascular disease. *Pakistan Journal of Medical Sciences*. 2014 Jan-Feb; 30(1): 194–197. doi:10.12669/pjms.301.4525

[3] Hu, J., La Vecchia, C., et al. (2011). Dietary transfatty acids and cancer risk. *European Journal of Cancer Prevention*. 2011 Nov;20(6):530-8. doi: 10.1097/CEJ.0b013e328348fbfb.

cause of deforestation in some countries in South East Asia, such as Indonesia and Malaysia. This is a major disaster, for several reasons:

- The loss of native forest. This releases carbon dioxide, and leaves us with fewer trees to soak up carbon dioxide, so it's a double whammy
- Destruction of peat bogs under those forests
- Loss of species biodiversity
- The Sumatran tiger faces imminent extinction
- Eventually, the orangutan faces extinction too, in the next decade

What do they use palm oil for? Well, most people are starting to know that palm oil is used in pastes, spreads, sauces and processed foods that need a certain consistency – things like chocolate spread, margarine, peanut butter and so on. But it turns out that estimates suggest as many as 75% of all the products in a modern supermarket have some amount of palm oil in them.

- Soaps and detergents
- Margarines and spreads
- Many breads, dough products (pizza bases, instant noodles, pastry cases, etc.)
- Cookies, ice creams, chocolate bars
- Cakes, pastries, pies, breakfast cereals, confectionery
- Washing powder
- Lipsticks, shower gels and other cosmetics
- Arguably, 'most' processed foods

There are many names for palm oil and its derivatives, too many to list. If you follow the MND way and stick to Core Principle 1 and 3, and cut the chemicals in Core Principle 4, you will be doing a pretty good job of reducing 90% of your palm oil consumption. When you do still purchase products with palm oil in them, try to look for a note on the label ensuring that the product uses sustainable palm oil.[4]

---

[4] WWF blog: *Palm reading: Should we buy or boycott products containing palm oil?* (2015, Nov 6). Retrieved from https://goo.gl/A1RcdK

Summary – the facts on fats

Let's keep the dietary science to a minimum. As I told you in 'My Story' way back at the start of this book, one of the things that pissed me off for two decades was trying to make sense of all the complicated science, conflicting evidence and confusion in the worlds of diet and nutrition. The last thing I want to do is make this book complex, overly-scientific or confusing. Most people just want to know "what should I eat to lose weight and stay healthy?" so I am trying to give you that as simply as possible.

Natural sources of good dietary fats are a healthy part of your diet[5]. Oily fish like salmon, tuna, sardines and mackerel, extra virgin olive oil and olives, nuts and seeds, avocados, free-range eggs, organic grass-fed meats, are all good healthy fats that you should enjoy in your diet.

Foods high in fat to include in a healthy diet:

- Oily fish
- Fish oils
- Avocado
- Extra virgin olive oil
- Olives
- Coconut oil
- Nuts and seeds
- Grass-fed meat and dairy
- Grass-fed butter
- Organic meat and dairy

---

[5] Malhotra, A., Redberg, R.F., & Meier, P. (2016). Saturated fat does not clog the arteries: coronary heart disease is a chronic inflammatory condition, the risk of which can be effectively reduced from healthy lifestyle interventions. *British Journal of Sports Medicine.* 2017;51:1111-1112. http://dx.doi.org/10.1136/bjsports-2016-097285

Fats to avoid in a healthy diet

- Trans fats
- Processed vegetable oils
- Processed seed oils
- Palm oil
- Margarines and spreads
- Grain-fed meat and dairy
- Cheap processed meat and dairy
- Processed foods that contain vegetable and seed oils, and palm oil, under its many names

What's the key message?

- Don't be afraid of fats if they are 'natural' – that means they come from fresh whole foods that have been raised to good ethical, organic standards, i.e. wild game or organic farmed meat and dairy, ideally 100% grass-fed. Enjoy good fats from foods such as olives, avocado, nuts, and fatty fish
- Best to largely avoid fats that have been processed – trans fats, palm oil, cheap processed vegetable oils and seed oils, as explained above
- Cook in butter or good lard. Good lard comes from roasting organic pork. Use extra virgin olive oil for cold dressings, such as on salads
- Coconut oil: sure, it's a good 'stable' fat to cook with, you can use that if you wish, but be wary not to get caught up in the hype of the 'latest trendy superfood'[6]
- Be aware of the calorie count of fats, especially snacking on nuts and seeds, those calories really can add up fast, a potential hazard if weight loss is your primary goal

---

[6] Of interest: https://www.abc.net.au/news/2019-03-02/super-foods-do-not-live-up-to-hype-say-qut-researchers/10847842

Core Principle 8

Animal rights matter. The environment matters. Human health, human rights, quality nutrition, animal welfare, farmer's welfare, the soil, the land, the seas and the air. Frankly, it all matters. If you think 'trying to do the right thing' just for health and weight loss is confusing, try **also** tying it all in with doing the right things for animal rights, farming standards and the environment too.

- I've spent twelve years doing just that
- It's a vast, complex and interconnected world
- The good news is, it's all covered in *Mother Nature's Diet* for you

Factory farms and caged animals

Modern industrialised agriculture is not good for food quality, not good for animal welfare and not good for the environment. **The advice in Core Principle 7 to 'eat plants and animals' comes hand-in-hand with Core Principle 8.** Quality matters. We should be looking to eat plants and animals that have themselves been raised on a healthy natural diet. We ideally want to eat plants that are local, seasonal and organic, and we want to eat animals that have been raised free-range, grazed on open pasture and treated humanely.

While humans are supposed to eat other animals, that does not give humans any right to shut those animals in a cage or mistreat those animals while they are alive. For better animal welfare, for better environmental management, for sustainability in farming, and for your health, we need to consume animal products that have come from animals which have lived as naturally as possible. We also want our plant foods free from man-made chemicals, many of which are toxic and may bio-accumulate inside our bodies.

Plants – local, seasonal, organic

In an ideal world, we want to eat vegetables and fruits grown as locally as possible. In recent years, we have all got used to having tropical fruits and summer fruits available all year-round in our supermarkets, but this comes at a cost, and it's the environment that is paying. There is a carbon footprint attached to eating bananas, strawberries and pineapples year-round in cold Northern Europe. Cutting a very, very long story short, we should ideally try to eat as much locally-grown produce as possible, and this will mean seasonal variations in our diet. Here in the UK, that's going to mean eating lots of those strawberries and raspberries in the spring and summer, but far fewer at other times of the year. More salads in summer, more hardy root vegetables in winter. Better for the environment, optimal for your health.

The best way to eat what is seasonally available is to learn to grow some of your own fruit and veg. Plant an apple tree, grow a few of your own cabbages or tomatoes, have a go at growing some strawberries, try to grow some lettuces in trays on your kitchen windowsill. You don't need much space, a few pots and planter trays will do, and you can start small and see how you get on.

Honestly, it really is easy. When I get new tyres put on our family car, I ask the mechanic to throw the old ones in the boot for me. I take them home, fill them with soil and compost and plant food in them. One courgette plant per tyre, takes five minutes to do, and it will grow huge! Try it. When you first taste your own home-grown food...oh wow, it's such an addictive hobby, it's so rewarding! If you are growing some of your own food, you will find it tastes fantastic, and you will know it is 100% organic, using no artificial chemicals at all.

Support local farmers

If you can, shop at a local farm shop or farmers market, try to support your local farming community. Engage with the sellers, ask if they are organic, how far the food has travelled.

While there is controversy around organic labelling, it still makes sense to go organic as much as you can afford. It is widely known and accepted that many pesticides are harmful to human health...but the argument goes, that by the time it is sprayed on crops, left to blow around in the wind, then the crop grows, then it is harvested, washed, transported and sold on...by the time each small individual piece of fruit or vegetable reaches you, then the residual small amount of pesticide left on that plant is so tiny, that any harmful effects are too small to worry about.

In essence, that argument is pretty logical and probably right. Your body is equipped to process some toxins and that one small meal with a tiny bit of pesticide residue in it really probably won't hurt you. But this seems to ignore the fact that you are going to eat more than one meal this year, aren't you? What this logic ignores, is the lifetime bio-accumulative[1] effect of eating about 1000 meals per year for 60 or 70 or 80 years. I really don't think they have done 70-year-long studies to look at that (we covered this back under Core Principle 4, on Page 111). They haven't done that research yet, but in my opinion, they really should. Bioaccumulation of POPs (Persistent Organic Pollutants[2]) is real, and studies link POPs in humans to cancer, heart disease and more.[3]

If you can afford to, just buy organic. The more we buy organic, the more the market will shift in the right direction and economies of scale will drive prices down.

In this book I have encouraged you to increase your vegetable and fruit consumption from the standard 5-a-day target, to 10 or 12 or 15 per day, or more! If you are doubling or tripling your vegetable intake, **those seemingly small amounts of pesticides are doubling or tripling too.** Now, it's the broccoli that might be killing you!! I'm serious!

It's time to buy organic!

If your budget is limited, then **buy organic** for the things where **you eat the outer surface** like broccoli, apples, grapes, spinach, tomatoes and strawberries. But things like pineapples, coconuts, melon, bananas and oranges, you peel and throw the skins away, so any pesticide residues on the skins are less of a worry. It's not 100% perfect, but it's a decent compromise. Remember one of our goals: progress, not perfection. Have you seen how often that keeps coming up? Words to live by, don't you think?

---

[1] Learn more: https://en.wikipedia.org/wiki/Bioaccumulation
[2] Learn more: https://en.wikipedia.org/wiki/Persistent_organic_pollutant
[3] Schafer, K.S., & Kegley, S.E. (2002). Persistent toxic chemicals in the US food supply. *BMJ. Journal of Epidemiology & Community Health*, 2002;56:813-817. https://jech.bmj.com/content/56/11/813

Animals – free range, grass fed, sustainably-caught

For animal welfare: Really, we have no right to dictate that any animal lives its life in a cage or box, all animals deserve to see day light and breathe fresh air, so let's just refuse to support farming that mistreats any animals. Enough said.

For human health: Ruminants (we're talking about cows and sheep here) are supposed to eat grass, not corn or soybeans, and the meat we get from those animals is healthier for us if they have been raised on a more natural diet. Grass-fed meat tends to be lower in omega-6 fatty acids and higher in omega-3 fatty acids than grain-fed meat, and this is beneficial for our health. Free range chickens produce healthier eggs. Sustainably-caught fish from the open ocean offer us better fats than farmed fish.

For the environment: Intensive, industrialised farming practises are not sustainable, and they are harmful to the topsoil, the air and to rivers and seas. This is a vast topic, that could easily fill an entire book on its own. I have researched the environmental impact of diets almost as much as I have research nutrition and health. I have spent years visiting farms, talking to farmers, attending agricultural conferences and reading books on soil fertility and greenhouse gases. To save *you* from *me* going off into that topic too deeply, I will keep this purposefully short! In very brief terms:

- Growing crops (such as corn, soybeans, wheat) to feed cows is a cause of deforestation and creates greenhouse gas emissions
- It's also an inefficient use of croplands and crops
- Cows should eat grass, not corn, soybeans or other grains!
- Trawling oceans for fish destroys marine life. Fish should be caught sustainably, by pole and line. Trawlers should be banned completely
- Intensive crop farming, focussed on the staples maize, wheat, soybeans, etc., causes fertilizer run-off which pollutes rivers and seas
- Intensive farming is depleting topsoil – yet free-ranged pastured cattle could be building topsoil, *and* locking up carbon from the atmosphere at the same time (now there is a hotly contested scientific topic right there!)

This chapter is purposefully brief. If you are interested in learning more about the environmental aspects of farming, I have written some good long blog posts[4] on the *Mother Nature's Diet* blog site[5] for you.[6] Please remember that Core Principle 7 and Core Principle 8 go hand-in-hand! For your health, for animal welfare, and for the sake of our environment. Let's do this thing right, let's be responsible global citizens, let's lead the way.

Key learning in this chapter

We want to eat plants and animals that have themselves been raised on a healthy natural diet. Trying to work out the perfect diet for weight loss and good health is **hard enough**, let alone trying to add in concerns for animal welfare, farming standards and saving the environment too! Lucky for you, *Mother Nature's Diet* is the place where all these things meet in the middle. 'Perfect' is **probably unachievable**, that's why we pursue progress, not perfection. When it comes to a healthy diet and lifestyle, healthy for us and healthy for the planet, MND gets as close as can be to the 'best of all worlds'.

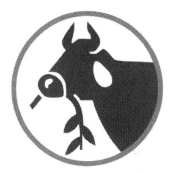

- We want to reduce our "lifetime load" exposure to pesticides, because many of the toxic compounds in pesticides bioaccumulate over time
- We want vegetables that have grown in fertile mineral-rich soils, because that makes for mineral-rich vegetables
- The best way to achieve these goals is to buy organic
- Even better, grow some of your own fruit and veg, it's fun, it saves you money and you get the best and freshest organic food possible
- Eat seasonally and buy local
- Frequent local farm shops and farmer's markets

---

4 *How intensive farming is causing greenhouse gas emissions.* See
https://mothernaturesdiet.me/2016/05/09/myth-busting-part-10/
5 *Why the answer is not just 'stop eating meat'.* See
https://mothernaturesdiet.me/2016/05/10/myth-busting-part-11/
6 *How grass-fed free-range ruminants can be the solution.* See
https://mothernaturesdiet.me/2016/05/11/myth-busting-part-12/

- If your budget is tight, opt organic for the things that you eat the 'outer surface' or skin, such as broccoli, apples, spinach, peaches, tomatoes, grapes
- Buy free-range and organic for animal welfare reasons. No excuses. Shop for quality, not quantity
- Buy grass-fed meat and dairy for a much healthier fatty acid composition in your food. For many of the reasons that I recommend humans shouldn't eat too many grains, so cows shouldn't eat all those grains either!
- Intensive, industrialised agriculture, plants and animals, is extremely environmentally destructive. It leads to deforestation, topsoil erosion, greenhouse gas emissions, river pollution and a loss of biodiversity on land and in the seas. If you care at all about the environment, opting for organic, sustainably-farmed, grass-fed and sustainably-caught fish, is a must
- Please always opt for sustainably-caught fish, look out for the MSC (Marine Stewardship Council) stamp as a mark of quality. Trawling is harmful to marine life, and harmful to the sea bed, and shop be stopped. If the damage trawler nets do was visible on land, it would be banned immediately

"We want to eat plants and animals that have themselves been raised on a healthy natural diet."

- And as for animal welfare, fish probably suffer more in being caught (they lay on deck and suffocate slowly, out of water, fully awake and conscious) than animals do in slaughter houses. Opting to be a vegetarian, but still eating fish, on grounds of animal welfare, makes no sense at all
- Shop for the best quality sustainably caught fish that you can afford, shop for local if you can

- Sure, everything covered in Core Principle 8 is going to push up your shopping budget by fifty quid or a hundred quid per month. Ask yourself, isn't it worth it? For better health? For animal welfare? For a better deal for farmers? To help halt climate change and biodiversity loss?
- Following MND you can easily save that money back – eat a bit less (focus on food quality, not quantity), **drink less booze**, give up satellite TV, grow your own veggies and you'll soon be saving far more than it costs you to buy organic and grass-fed

You can use this page for your own notes.

Core Principle 9

If we had to summarise the *Mother Nature's Diet* approach to exercise in a 'one size fits all' approach (which of course, it doesn't!) then it might be to make these five simple statements: 1: Go for a walk every day. 2: Two or three times per week do some exercise that pushes your heart rate up, makes your lungs work and gets you sweating. 3: Also, two or three times each week, do some strength exercise to stimulate your muscles, and don't neglect this as you get older – in many respects, the older you get, the more important strength training becomes!

And then 4: Beyond that, live a full and active life, stay busy, and don't spend hours or days on end sitting down. 5: The secrets to success in activity and exercise are consistency and variety. It's not what you do once in a while that defines you, it's what you do habitually, daily, that leads to progress.

Use it or lose it

Your body is the most amazing thing you will ever own – **use it or lose it.** That applies to fitness, strength and flexibility (...and your brain, and also your sex life!)

I would strongly recommend you re-read those last two lines about fifty times, think about it, really let that sink in. What you don't use, for years, you will lose. As you age, if you let your fitness go, chances are it'll be gone for good. If you let your strength go, every likelihood is, it'll be gone for good. If you let your flexibility go, you'll struggle to ever get it back. **Is that what you want?**

Really think about that. Ageing is what you make it. You can buy-in to the story that your fitness and strength decline as you age, or you can resolve to work hard to stay in good shape. **You have a choice.** Personally, as I write this, I am approaching 50 years of age, and through my 40s I've been in the best shape of my life, and I'm still working on getting better.

You have to move: get off your butt

There's not an animal on the planet that doesn't move. There isn't one. There's not an animal on the planet that lives an entirely sedentary lifestyle. Humans are the same, we have evolved to be active. You have to move. According to Cancer Research UK, being inactive and a lack of exercise is the fifth leading preventable cause of cancer in the UK, and causes around 1% to 2% of UK cancers. Lack of exercise can be a contributing factor in breast cancer, bowel cancer and womb cancer. Remember, it's a key theme of this whole book, **you have a choice.**

According to the NHS, regular exercise is one of the best ways you can protect yourself from heart disease. The NHS states *"Step right up! It's the miracle cure we've all been waiting for. It can reduce your risk of major illnesses, such as heart disease, stroke, type 2 diabetes and cancer by up to 50% and lower your risk of early death by up to 30%. It's free, easy to take, has an immediate effect and you don't need a GP to get some. Its name? Exercise."*[1] Heart disease and cancer, Britain's two biggest killers right there. You've got to develop a daily exercise habit.

First steps: be active

It's worth taking a moment to differentiate between exercise, and activity.

Exercise: we are talking about purposeful structured movement that you do for the benefits of fun, burning calories, relieving stress, getting stronger, sculpting your body and so on. This includes things like going running, playing a sport you enjoy, swimming, lifting weights, riding your bike, doing push-ups, building muscle and so on. Gym sessions and runs and workouts on the living room floor are examples of exercise.

Activity: On the other hand, when we talk about activity, we are talking about the movements you do every day as part of your ordinary life – walking up the stairs, carrying bags, working, shopping, walking your dog, doing the

---

[1] NHS website, *Benefits of Exercise*, see https://www.nhs.uk/live-well/exercise/exercise-health-benefits/

school run, having sex, popping out to post a letter or get something from the local shops, visiting friends, mowing the lawn, washing the car and painting the spare room. All these little daily chores, and our work, are examples of activity.

Shift your mindset around exercise

There are many good reasons to exercise, and I am going to cover most of them in this chapter, but one of the main reasons why many people engage in exercise is to 'fight the fat' and lose unwanted weight. However, in truth, exercise is actually not particularly good at doing that!

Now before you give up, let me explain! I believe we should all aim to exercise every day, because of the many benefits of exercise, and because it's fun and it makes you feel good, and because a consistent daily exercise habit certainly does help, combined with a healthy diet, in weight loss and body shaping. But the reality is that the actual number of calories you burn in a structured exercise session is really not that great. People think that they can exercise the pounds away, but in fact you'll find getting your diet right is far more beneficial than doing loads of exercise.

In general, when people do 'small to modest' amounts of exercise, they only burn relatively small amounts of calories. An hour of average-intensity mixed activity in a typical commercial gym, perhaps consisting of 20 minutes on a sit-down exercise bike and then a few circuits of the resistance machines, for a 140-pound (10 stone) woman of 50, will likely only really burn a few hundred calories at most, about the equivalent of one moderate lunch of a big salad and a piece of chicken.

And if the exercise session is a big one, like two hours out running a half marathon or something like that, then yes that does burn a more appreciable number of calories, but all too often the person then *feels* they have worked really hard, they are exhausted and starving, and they eat extra calories to compensate! As a retired marathon runner myself, with many runner friends, I see this literally all the time. Folks put in a big session and then reward themselves with pizza and ice cream!

I am not trying to put you off exercise! This chapter is all about the benefits of exercise, and it certainly does play a helpful role in weight management, but understand that activity is more important than exercise when it comes to weight loss. Also, you have to know that the saying "You can't outrun a bad diet" is absolutely true.

When it comes to weight loss, our first goal should be activity, and then exercise. Activity (it's known as NEAT in the exercise business – Non-Exercise Activity Thermogenesis – meaning the calories you burn from activity other than structured exercise sessions) is your friend, and a lifestyle that is busy and active and involves lots of time on your feet and moving, will likely burn far more calories for you every day and every week, than those 40- to 50-minute jogs and gym sessions that you've been told are so important.

Once you have your active lifestyle in place, then exercise should be seen as a 'tool' you can use, when required, rather than an end-goal in and of itself. Exercise is good for your heart, can help prevent disease, can help resist ageing and can shape and sculpt your body – but if weight loss is your number one goal, then you need to remember that day-to-day activity is probably more important than exercise. Our goals should be to be active and moving lots every day, to spend time outdoors, to be playing, having fun, having sex, enjoying life and keeping busy.

If you can get enough daily activity from walking every day, playing games and sports that you enjoy, and enjoying an active sex life, and doing all your daily chores like your work and growing some of our own food in the garden, then you can treat structured exercise simply as a 'supplement to a busy life' to shape certain body parts and achieve specific strength and fitness outcomes.

Activity is your friend, and a lifestyle that is busy and active and involves lots of time on your feet and moving, will **likely burn far more calories** for you every day and every week, than those 40- to 50-minute jogs and gym sessions that you've been told are so important.

Once you have your active lifestyle in place, then exercise should be seen as a tool you can use, when required, rather than an end-goal in and of itself.

Exercise is good for **your heart**, can help **prevent disease**, can help **resist ageing** and can shape and **sculpt your body** – but if weight loss is your #1 goal, then you need to remember that overall, day-to-day activity is probably more important than exercise.

Move naturally

If you're interested, there's a fantastic book titled *Blue Zones*, by a guy called Dan Buettner. Of those 847 books I have read on health, nutrition and disease prevention, this is absolutely one of my personal favourites, and it's probably the single book I recommend more often than any other. If you're not into reading books (FGS, what's wrong with you???), just watch his inspired and captivating 20-minute TED talk[2] instead, it is so very well worth watching. This guy and his team from National Geographic went around the world for several years meeting and studying people who live to extraordinary old age. They met wonderful 108-year-old Japanese grandmas and Sardinian shepherds who enjoy fantastic good health in their 90s and 100s, and they spent years studying them, taking blood samples, watching them, tracking their diets, and learning about how they use their bodies.

If you watch that TED talk, you'll see at 15 minutes in, Dan starts to summarise the nine key things they learned researching and writing the book. These nine factors make the summary chapters in the book. The number one factor they found all these people had in common, was **'move naturally'**. All these people, in diverse communities around the world, had this one thing in common above all others. Hardly any of them engaged in structured, purposeful exercise, but without exception they all led busy active lives, **they all walked a lot, usually on hills**, and they all kept busy using their bodies for work and chores – lifting, shifting, carrying and working on through their 80s, 90s and 100s.

The message: stay active, and walk every day.
Use your body.

Benefits of cardiovascular exercise

Just as all the reports and studies and books on nutrition and diet are conflicting and confusing, so it is with exercise! For decades the standard advice was to avoid eating fat and base your diet on starchy carbohydrates,

---

[2] TED talks: *How to live to be 100+.* (2009, Sept). Retrieved from https://www.ted.com/talks/dan_buettner_how_to_live_to_be_100#t-954329

and at the same time the so-called experts of their day told everyone to go jogging and join an aerobics class!

Now the advice says it's the sugar and carbs all along that's been making us fat, and that all that jogging is ruining your knees and what you should all be doing is weight training! OMG, how the heck can the general public be expected to trust any of these people!!! They gave us all the wrong advice for 40 years – maybe now this is the wrong advice again?!?!?

Once again, *Mother Nature's Diet* to the rescue. Remember my story, my journey, I have been through it all, the running, the injuries, the knee surgery. I'm a qualified Personal Trainer, I cycle, lift weights, run, go rock climbing; I've done it all and read hundreds of books and sorted out all the science for you. Let's get to the facts in short and simple form:

- Studies prove that there are life-extending benefits to engaging in cardiovascular exercise. [3] Cardiovascular exercise is things like running, cycling and swimming, stuff that gets your heart rate elevated, gets you puffing and panting and sweating

- Cardiovascular exercise is essential for a healthy heart and helps us to live longer[4]

- Studies seem to show that endurance athletes live a little longer than the average population (about two to four years longer, but research results vary), most likely because of the cardiovascular benefits for their hearts (remember that heart disease is the global #1 killer)

- More is not necessarily better. While moderate amounts of cardiovascular exercise are shown to confer benefits, extreme amounts of additional exercise do not confer any greater benefits. In other words, if you go from sedentary, to exercising once per week, then from once per week to twice per week, then from twice per week to three times per week, each step of the way shows benefits to your health and additional protection from heart disease. But this

---

[3] Hirsch, C.H., Diehr, P., et al (2010). Physical Activity and Years of Healthy Life in Older Adults: Results From the Cardiovascular Health Study. *Journal of Aging and Physical Activity.* 2010 Jul; 18(3): 313–334. Retrieved from https://www.ncbi.nlm.nih.gov/pmc/articles/PMC3978479/

[4] Birkenhäger, W.H., de Leeuw, P.W., (2002). 'Survival of the fittest': effect of regular physical exercise on health and life expectancy. *Ned Tijdschr Geneeskd.* 2002 Aug 10;146(32):1479-83. Retrieved from https://www.ncbi.nlm.nih.gov/pubmed/12198825

progression stops at 'moderate' amounts of exercise. If you go from a 30- or 40-minute run three times per week, up to an hour-long run six times per week, you gain very little, if any, additional benefits
- Worse, all that additional exercise, depending on how you run, your technique, natural gait, shoes, terrain, bodyweight, and more, may possibly place demands on your knees and hips that could lead to injuries

And that's how we reach the *Mother Nature's Diet* conclusion – engage in cardiovascular exercise two or three times per week. Aim for consistency and variety.

- Consistency = make it a habit for life, a couple of times per week forever
- Variety = mix things up, go for some variety. A run one day, a bike ride another time, maybe go swimming, try a rowing machine when you are in the gym. Variety is good, it helps prevent repetitive strain injuries from always doing the same thing

"You have two legs and one arse, I suggest you use them in that proportion!"

Aim to spend twice as much time on your feet as you do on your butt, that's going to be a major step in the right direction.

Benefits of strength training

One of the most commonly-accepted measures of ageing is frailty. Frailty is ageing. Ageing is frailty. We've all met the 60-year old who seems worn out and ready to drop, and we've all met the 90-year old who seems full of beans and making plans for the future. You see, the number of candles on your cake may tell us your age, but it is not a reliable measure of how well you are ageing.

Frailty, however, is. Once a person becomes frail, it's the beginning of the end.

- When you can no longer stand up from the toilet without grab handles or assistance, that's frailty
- When you can't step over the side of the bath unassisted for fear of falling, that's frailty
- When you can't get the lid off the jar anymore, maybe you can't prepare your own food any longer, and you need to move into assisted living
- When you no longer have the strength to pick up a full kettle of boiling water without dropping it and possibly scalding yourself, you're not safe in your own kitchen anymore, then it's time for the old folks' home
- When you are scared of walking down the street because a trip may mean a fall and a broken hip, that's frailty

Loss of strength, loss of muscle, is key to ageing.[5] If you're 45 reading this, maybe you think it all seems a way off, but ask yourself how much has your strength declined from 25 to 45? If it does the same from 45 to 65, where will that leave you? You have to use your muscles a couple of times per week to maintain that strength.

Remember: use it or lose it.

This advice, to engage in some strength training at least a couple of times per week, this applies more to the 50-year old woman reading this, than it does to the 30-year old man. Chances are the 30-year old man who buys this book already goes to a gym and uses weights, or he already plays some sport regularly, or he already works on strength training every week. It's the 50-year old woman who is most at risk of losing her strength. That's not being

---

[5] Syddall, H., et al, (2003) Is grip strength a useful single marker of frailty? *Age and Ageing*, Volume 32, Issue 6, 1 November 2003, Pages 650–656, https://doi.org/10.1093/ageing/afg111

sexist, ageist or meaning to cast broad judgements, it's just the facts I have observed in my experience over a number of years. **Ladies, please, go lift.**[6]

Aside from ageing...

Beyond the benefits or resisting the onset of frailty, there are so many more good reasons to enjoy strength training a couple of times every week:

- Strength training is an essential part of being human. Maintaining our muscular strength as we age helps us remain youthful and is a proven anti-ageing strategy – not just resisting frailty as we have covered, but in retaining our abilities to function in all areas of life – in work and in play
- Strong is sexy!
- Muscle helps to burn calories. Unlike fat, muscle is biologically active, so it helps your body to burn calories all day long, even while you sleep. The numbers aren't huge, but every little helps
- Maintaining our strength helps to keep us free from injuries, it stabilises our joints and protects us from falls and sprains
- Muscle shapes our bodies in desirable ways (fat tends to shape our bodies in undesirable ways)
- Studies suggest that strength training helps us to live longer[7]
- Weight training is fun. Really, lifting those weights can feel surprisingly satisfying. If you have never tried it...go on, you might just find you enjoy it!

Studies seem to show that extreme strength athletes live slightly shorter lives than the general population, though there is conflicting evidence here. It seems there are **no disadvantages** to moderate amounts of strength training,

---

[6] Kamada, M., Shiroma, E.J., et al, (2017). Strength Training and All-Cause, Cardiovascular Disease, and Cancer Mortality in Older Women: A Cohort Study. *Journal of the American Heart Association*, 6(11), 31-Oct-2017. doi: 10.1161/JAHA.117.007677
[7] British Journal of Sports Medicine blog: *Resistance training – an underutilised drug available in everybody's medicine cabinet.* (2017, Nov 27). Retrieved from https://blogs.bmj.com/bjsm/2017/11/27/resistance-training-underutilised-drug-available-everybodys-medicine-cabinet/

only advantages, but perhaps there are *some* disadvantages to the *extreme end* of the spectrum. (It's worth noting that so far, the science is all pretty mixed and inconclusive.) So, my advice would be to use your muscles, do some strength training a couple of times per week, but try to avoid becoming the seven-days-per-week gym addict, high-intensity weight lifter or monster-size-is-all-that-matters bodybuilder, as taking strength training to these extremes can possibly become counter-productive from a health standpoint.

Bodyweight training at home

There are many ways to train for strength. A lot of folks assume that lifting weights in a gym full of muscle-bound young hunks is your only option. That may or may not sound appealing to you! In fact, if you don't fancy the gym environment then you might like to try training at home.

You could try mostly body-weight moves, or add some cheap home workout gear you can buy online, like hand weights, a resistance band, or a kettlebell. It's easier than you might think to set up at home, just clear a little space, perhaps put down a yoga mat for grip, and you might like to crank up some music. You can do some push-ups, crunches, squats, lift weights over your head and try a variety of jumps and lunges and so on.

There is not space in this book to start explaining how to do lots of exercises and set out too many workouts (you'll find a few basic ideas in the 28-Day Plan), I just want you to see that when I suggest you "work your muscles a couple of times per week" that does not mean you *must* join a gym, dress head-to-foot in Lycra and start pumping iron in the quest for the body beautiful.

If you want to do that, then that's great, but you don't *have* to. You may work your muscles a few times per week by devising a nice little home workout routine including a few squats, lunges, crunches, push-ups, curls and shoulder presses. If you don't know how to do these moves, you can just search "How to do a ..." and the name of the move into *YouTube* and you'll quickly find a dozen free demonstrations to show you how it's done.

The point is, anyone can clear a little space, buy a yoga mat and a couple of little hand weights for about twenty-five quid, and then make time to work through your 15- or 20-minute routine three times a week. It's not that hard. Where there's a will, there's a way.

Remember – progress, not perfection. That's the goal here. We want to get you using your muscles, retaining your strength as you age, for so many good reasons. You can fit your training in while you are out too, in the park while you are out for a jog or a walk. I do that all the time. Chin-ups on tree branches, push-ups in the park, and dips on park benches. Maybe your chosen sport uses your muscles. You could go and have fun on an indoor climbing wall, that's a great upper-body-strength workout. Take a weekly yoga class, or Pilates, or join a gym class swinging kettlebells or a 'bootcamp' class flipping tractor tyres. There are many ways to train for strength; I encourage you to find one you enjoy.

Navigating the confusion

There is a shocking amount of bad information out there when it comes to exercise, weight loss and what is healthy for your body. It would be easy to believe that having a rippling 6-pack is the ultimate symbol of a healthy body; that we should all be drinking proteins shakes every day; and that you can't possibly run properly without a £130 pair of gel running shoes.

But actually, there is no science whatsoever to substantiate any of that. The reality is, that studies show 'pinch an inch' is probably actually a little **healthier** that 'rippling 6-pack abs'; and guzzling protein shakes will probably cause many people gastrointestinal distress before it helps them build big muscles; and once you learn to run properly in ways that don't trash your knees, then it doesn't really matter that much what shoes you wear to do it.

- Don't believe the hype, most of these workout programs, 6-pack solutions, endless online programs and routines are little more than modern solutions, to a modern problem, called sedentary lifestyles, and they will shrink your bank account as quickly as your waistline, or quicker
- Longevity is a vital element of the MND lifestyle. Ageing doesn't have a brake pedal, only an accelerator. Try not to spend your life pushing down too hard on that accelerator. That 18-stone bodybuilder eating 7000 calories per day is pushing way too hard
- Working out too hard or too much, all the time, is almost certainly counter-productive to your health objectives
- Regular, long, brisk (and hilly) walks are probably just about the best fat burning exercise we can possibly do, and they get you out in nature, and they are fun, and they give you fresh air, and you can share with a friend or loved one, and they get you away from your TV or computer – what's not to love!

Stretch

Stretch often; keep your body supple and mobile. Avoid injuries, look after your structure and see an osteopath if you need help with your posture. Once you lose your flexibility, if you're in your 50s or 60s, oh boy then it's hard to get it back. Stretch, a couple of times per week. Look after your spine, and your knees. You want those joints to last you a long time.

Summary: Core Principle 9 – Exercise!

Phew! It's been another fairly big chapter, well done for sticking it out, good for you! I will keep this summary short and to the point. Exercise and activity are super important. You cannot ignore the proven health benefits of being active.[8] Build more activity in to your life. You can park 20 minutes away from work and take a brisk walk in and then a brisk walk back at the end of the day. See how easy that is? Entirely sedentary people die younger than people who exercise regularly. **That's insane! Ignoring exercise can cost you years off your life!**

"You won't shape an amazing butt by sitting on it!"

Try to ensure your typical week includes a walk almost every day, a couple of cardio sessions, a couple of strength sessions and some stretching. Learn to use your own bodyweight for strength training – you can be your own gym, any time, any place! Consistency is key! Make exercise habits that you can stick to for life. It's better to exercise for half an hour, five days per week, and stick to it all year, than to be all 'Mr-20-hours-per-week' down the gym for a month and then quit for the rest of the year. Consistency is key.

---

[8] American Psychological Association. (2009, Aug 10). Sedentary Lives Can Be Deadly: Physical Inactivity Poses Greatest Health Risk To Americans, Expert Says. *ScienceDaily*. Retrieved from www.sciencedaily.com/releases/2009/08/090810024825.htm

- Use it or lose it; you have to move
- Be active. If weight loss is your goal, activity and a good diet are your best friends
- Move naturally. Walk every day, and use your body for work and play
- The biggest killer in our society is heart disease – get some cardiovascular exercise a couple of times a week for heart health and circulation
- Folks who do their cardio, live longer. Fact
- You have two legs and one arse, I suggest you use them in that proportion
- Lift some weights, or at least your own bodyweight
- The benefits of strength training are numerous, particularly as you get older, they help stave off frailty, the key marker of ageing
- You won't shape an amazing butt by sitting on it
- Get up, get off the sofa, hit the gym
- Stretch often, take up yoga, maintain your flexibility and range-of-motion
- Ignoring the advice in this chapter could cost you several years off your life, that's a really big deal, that's as serious as smoking or being diagnosed diabetic. No excuses, you have to exercise
- Consistency is king. Find what you enjoy, do it every week. For life

"Be active! Exercise, every day, outdoors, mostly walking. Lift some heavy things and use your muscles a few times each week, and sprint from time to time. Stretch often and don't become a crazy exercise addict!"

You can use this page for your own notes.

Core Principle 10

C hronic lifestyle stress is more of a burden than most of us realise. Chronic stress is a major cause of ill health, yet it's something we have come to live with, as a society, and we rarely even seem to question it these days. The 15-hour work days that people seem to boast about like it's some 'badge of honour', the constant tiredness, the debt and money worries – it's almost become that you are weird if you don't have these issues, they have become the new norm. This is not good.

Stress drains your energy, it makes your body hold on to fat, and it kills your libido. If you eat a good diet and exercise but you still can't lose that excess 20 pounds, it might be that stress reduction is a big part of the answer. If you are healthy, active and successful in business but you wonder where your sex life has gone, it might be that stress is the problem. Many experts agree that stress is a major

contributor to lifestyle diseases, such as heart disease and cancer. Two or three decades of constant low-level stress can be very harmful. Get a handle on things now and manage your life more effectively to reduce the stress burden on your health.

In a nutshell: Chronic stress is bad for you. That's everything from ringing alarm clocks interrupting your much-needed sleep and day-to-day hassles and worries, to bankruptcy, divorce and career pressure. This is the stuff we often live with for decades on end, and it all has a negative impact on our health. Many studies link stress to many major illnesses, including the big killers – heart disease[1], cancer, diabetes and obesity. We want to reduce

---

[1] British Heart Foundation: *Feeling stressed? Research shows how stress can lead to heart attacks and stroke.* (2017). Retrieved from https://www.bhf.org.uk/informationsupport/heart-matters-magazine/news/behind-the-headlines/stress-and-heart-disease

stress, love more, smile more often, have less debt, get more sleep and enjoy life. Happy is healthy, and vice versa. Stress is such a big deal, that any so-called diet book or health book that doesn't address stress reduction, sleep quality and relaxation, in my opinion isn't worth the paper it's printed on. Let's work through Core Principle 10 and see how it all fits together.

Core Principle 10: Reduce stress. Enjoy your life. Love more, don't hate. Sleep, relax, smile, pray

Reduce stress

This is another one of those topics that could fill an entire book, or several, all on its own. (Yeah, I know, the 12 Core Principles could easily fill 12 books...) We want to keep this brief, and not get lost in too much science, so if you'll forgive me, I will just dump a couple of nuggets of information on you, and we'll stop short of delving deep into the how and why it all works the way it works.

It's all about your hormones

Everything in the human body interacts with everything else. There is virtually no system or function that operates in isolation, everything is interconnected by your central nervous system (kinda like the wiring in your supercomputer), your blood (the river of life) and by the chemical signals and instructions that blood carries around, in the form of hormones, proteins and other compounds.

Hormones arrive at an organ or a certain type of tissue or cell, and deliver instructions telling those tissues or cells what to do. When hormone signalling works well, like signalling in a computer or on a railway network, all is well. When signalling is 'shot to shit', just like on a road or rail network, all hell breaks loose, and we either have major crashes, or everything seizes up in grid lock. That's how important hormones are.

You have hormones that govern when you feel hungry or full; hormones that make you happy or sad, angry or calm, lively or relaxed. Hormones and minerals between them regulate many complex processes in the body including appetite, blood pressure and elimination of waste.

Fight or flight...rest and digest

You have likely heard of the 'fight or flight' response. When you feel fear, when you sense some imminent danger, your body releases a rush of stress hormones (adrenaline and cortisol are the ones you will have heard of) and prepare you to either fight, physically, or to run away. Yes, this all dates back to caveman and the proverbial sabre-toothed tiger; these hormonal systems have been keeping us safe since our ancient ancestors climbed down out of the trees in East Africa around seven million years ago.

The opposite 'hormonal state' to **fight or flight**, is **'rest and digest'**. At any time, your body can be in one or the other state, but it can't do both at the same time, as they are polar opposites. When you are in stress response mode, fight or flight, and those stress hormones flood your body, they trigger a whole bunch of things to happen. They divert your body's energy resources away from things like 'fighting off the common cold' and 'digesting breakfast' and 'making my hair nice and shiny' in favour of more immediately useful functions like 'run like hell' and 'fight the tiger/wrestle the alligator' and so on. In effect, what this means is, a flood of stress hormones shuts down your immune system, your digestive system and your anti-ageing, beauty systems, in favour of stuff that's going to keep you alive for the next ten minutes – the ability to fight, grapple and run. You feel awake, alert, strong...but inside, other systems have been put on hold temporarily for you to feel that way.

Now, can you see, that if you spend half your life living in a stress response, then you spend half your life with compromised immune function, compromised digestive function and compromised anti-ageing functions?

Now you can see, how 30 years of chronic stress can lead to:

- Poor immune function – catch coughs and colds all the time
- Poor immune function long term – increased risk of cancer and heart disease
- Poor digestive function – IBS, bloating, gas, diarrhoea, constipation, poor absorption of minerals and other nutrients
- Weak anti-ageing systems – 'look like shit', bad skin, hair, nails

Chronic stress, through hormone havoc, takes a toll. In broad terms, hormonally, the opposite bodily state to fight or flight, is rest and digest. Now that makes sense, doesn't it? You can see how we evolved such systems millions of years ago. There are times we need to be ready to fight, or take flight, such as out on the hunt, and then there are times we can rest, and divert our body's energy to digestion and immune function, such as when we are relaxed around the comparative safety of the camp fire.

Biologically, you can't do both at once. It's black and white. North and South. They are opposites. You can't do both at the same time.

Now you know why they say you shouldn't eat when you are in a highly agitated state, when you are totally stressed out. It's because digestive processes require vast amounts of your body's energy – to produce stomach acid, without which you will not digest proteins properly; to power peristaltic action, moving your food down through your bowels ready for elimination; to increase blood flow around the gut, ready to take the nutrients from your food and move them to your liver and from there off all around your body.

You see, digestion takes a lot of energy (that's why you feel sleepy after a big meal) and your body cannot be on high alert, ready to fight, if all that energy is working on digestion. So, when the alert signal comes (when stress hormones are released), blood flow is diverted away from the gut and sent to the muscles instead, and digestive function is temporarily compromised.

And we are not even starting to talk about many of the subtler nuances here. In 'fight or flight' your body is trying to raise blood sugar, to fuel your muscles...in 'rest and digest' your body is trying to lower blood sugar, as part of the natural 'digest and file away nutrients' process of replenishment. There are many such processes that we don't have space to go in to here.

"Digestion takes a lot of energy (that's why you feel sleepy after a big meal)"

In broad terms, hormonally, the opposite bodily state to **fight or flight**, is **rest and digest**. Now that makes sense, doesn't it? You can see how we evolved such systems millions of years ago. There are times we need to be ready to fight, or take flight, such as out on the hunt, and then there are times we can rest, and divert our body's energy to digest, such as when we are relaxed around the safety of the camp fire.

Biologically, you can't do both at once. It's black and white. North and South. They are opposites. You can't do both at the same time.

HPA axis dysfunction

All this 'hormone havoc' builds up over time, and if it goes on for years, you can end up with something called HPA axis dysfunction. Honestly, it's about as complicated as human biology gets, and I am not going to delve into it here, this book is not a science book, I am trying to keep this to 'easy-reading' if I can. If you want to understand HPA axis dysfunction, try a Google search, and good luck, it's a rabbit hole you may be down for a long time.

The upshot is, that chronic HPA axis dysfunction is implicated in obesity, type-2 diabetes, heart disease and stroke, cancer, sleep disturbance, cognitive decline, and just about 90% of everything else that goes wrong with human bodies and eventually kills us. If I had to answer "How do you fix it?" in one sentence, I would say "Reduce stress, get more sleep, learn to love, relax and smile a lot more." Ummm, sounds a lot like **Core Principle 10** of *Mother Nature's Diet*, don't you think?

Lifestyle stress

I hope I have given you enough detail to convince you that a lifetime of stress over work and money, just to die 15 years prematurely and leave that expensive German-made car on your driveway, is not worth it.

The big areas that cause stress in our modern Western culture are work, money, debt and relationships. We tend to get ourselves bogged down in stress over money – earning it, spending it, and never having enough of it. Ironically, the one thing you can't buy is good health, yet so many people are harming their own good health in the pursuit of money, to buy things that actually don't do much to make their lives substantially happier.

Enjoy your work. If you don't, change your job. Don't get trapped in the cycle of working a job you don't enjoy, to service high debts, to own stuff that doesn't ultimately make you happy. It is just a pointless way to live your life. **Buy less, live within your means, do a job you enjoy, relax more often.**

Stop borrowing, stop over-spending. So many people just can't get their brain around this. Let's say you earn 30, then you need to learn to live on 28. It's called **saving!** Put the 'two spare' away, and after a few years, you can invest your savings in something that will give you a return, such as your pension, or a spare property, or stocks. Do this throughout your whole life, and you will be able to live very comfortably in older age.

The trouble is, far too many folks out there earn 30, and live a lifestyle that costs 32. They do this using credit cards, car loans, overdrafts, bank loans, mortgages and more. They do this for decades on end, then have to keep borrowing against the equity in their home to cover their debts. This causes relationship strain, arguments, and lots of stress. Too many folks do this their whole lives and then wind up broke at retirement age. **It's a stupid way to live. Just stop it and live within your means!**

If you stop over-spending, and develop the habit of spending a little less than you earn, and saving a little each month, then some time down the line, when things go wrong, you might just find that you have enough reserves in place to cover the challenges of life without them becoming too much of a drama. If you put these good habits in place when you are young, in your 20s or 30s, by the time you are in your 50s and 60s, **life will feel much easier.** The problem is, far too many folks don't work this stuff out until they are hitting retirement age.

Time to work on the solution

We've established that stress is very unhealthy. Personally, I think it is at least as significant as whether or not you smoke, drink heavily or take regular exercise.

If you are slim, lean, you eat your 5-a-day and you don't smoke, and you exercise a couple of times per week, you might think all this health advice malarkey isn't for you. Oh yes it is! I've got news for you – **slim people die too!** Lean people get cancer too. Non-smokers die too you know.

NEWS FLASH – being slim doesn't mean you're gonna live forever! Honestly, truly, I'm sorry to be the miserable bastard to break it to you, I really am, but the truth is that there is no single magic bullet. We have all met the slim, non-smoker, who kept active and didn't drink much but still got breast cancer at 54. We've all heard of the business man who didn't smoke, ran the London 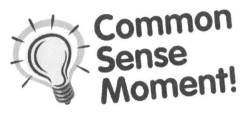 marathon every year and was always bright and smiling, yet keeled over with a massive heart attack at just 58.

I'm sorry folks but these things happen. Being slim doesn't mean you're going to live forever, being a non-smoker isn't the single magic bullet solution to living to 95 in perfect good health. As you will understand by the time you get to the end of this book, the causes of cancer, heart disease, stroke and most other life-ending conditions are multifactorial, complex, and very often individual. **One size does not fit all.**

All the factors we discuss in this book matter. People who are not overweight but still eat a lot of sugar, more often than not suffer the same metabolic problems (insulin resistance being the main one) that overweight sugar-eaters suffer too. Someone who is overweight or obese, but exercises regularly and keeps fit, is likely to live longer and in better health than someone slim who takes no exercise and is not at all fit. That's a hard truth for a lot of people to handle, but it's backed up by science. Fitness actually matters more than fatness.[2]

There are many factors at play, which explains why one size does not fit all, and why science doesn't yet have all the answers. If it really was as simple as "eat broccoli three times a week and you won't get cancer" then some clever PhD would have told us by now and claimed themselves a Nobel prize along the way. If it was as simple as "exercise regularly and you are guaranteed to never have a heart attack" then every government and health authority around the world would encourage its population to exercise regularly...

Oh, hang on a minute...you might want to check what it says on the NHS website about that...under the headline 'Benefits of exercise'. Here, allow me to share the first few lines with you...

---

[2] Mother Nature's Diet blog: *Fitness or fatness?* (2016, Dec 7) Read more: https://mothernaturesdiet.me/2016/12/07/fitness-or-fatness/

Quoting directly from the NHS website:[3]

> **"Step right up! It's the miracle cure we've all been waiting for.**
>
> It can reduce your risk of major illnesses, such as heart disease, stroke, type 2 diabetes and cancer by up to 50% and lower your risk of early death by up to 30%.
>
> It's free, easy to take, has an immediate effect and you don't need a GP to get some. Its name? Exercise."

The causes of ill health are complex, and the causal factors stack one on top of the other, increasing your risks of type-2 diabetes, heart disease and cancer as you go.

- Genetics matter too (but not as much as you might think)
- Stress matters too (likely far more than you think)
- Sleep matters too (it's the quickest and easiest 'cure' for too much stress, just get more sleep)

And so that brings us to the rest of MND Core Principle 10: **Enjoy your life. Love more, don't hate. Sleep, relax, smile, pray.** The best antidote to all this chronic stress is to get more sleep and spend more time relaxing. Meditate daily, get some exercise, ensure every day includes a little time outside getting some fresh air and as often as possible, some sunshine.

- Enjoy your life
- Laugh more often, make time to play, enjoy comedy and have more fun
- Be adaptable, be flexible, and be forgiving. Be kind to other people
- Take a day off. Stop and smell the roses

---

[3] See 'Benefits of Exercise': https://www.nhs.uk/live-well/exercise/exercise-health-benefits/

- Love more, don't hate
- The world needs more love, and less hate and resentment. Negative emotions are costly, they cost you your health. It's just not worth holding on to anger, bitterness or resentment. Let go, it's wreaking havoc with your hormones and costing you dearly. Someone wiser than me once said "No thought lives in your head rent free."
- Sleep more
- Regular good quality sleep is probably your best weapon against chronic stress. Aim for seven to eight hours per night – maybe more if you are an athlete
- Keep your bed for sleep, making love, and reading. Nothing else. No food in bed, no TV in bed, leave your laptop, tablet and smartphone out of reach
- You should sleep in proper darkness – no night lights, no red standby lights on electronic devices, no checking your smartphone when you wake up to pee in the middle of the night; get some good thick curtains
- Smile, and laugh, and try to bring happiness into your life
- We used to think that smiling was the end product of happy emotions in the brain, but some clever researchers did a series of studies where they wired up people's brains and they had them sitting there completely neutral, and then they said, "Smile." When the people were forced to smile, the pleasure sensors in the brain lit up. In other words, it works both ways. Smiling can be both cause, and effect. You smile when you feel happy, but you can make yourself feel happy, by smiling. If you're feeling down, stand up, breathe, get some fresh air, move, and smile, and you will feel better
- Cheer up, decide to be a happy person, life is amazing, but it's all-too-often not long enough, so make the most of every day
- Seriously, happiness really is 'an inside job', so get to it, and don't delay!
- Develop a positive outlook on life. Frankly, in the lottery of life, we are absolute winners. This is the UK, it's the 21st century. We've never had it so good. Know that, and celebrate it every day
- Know that 'shit happens' and that's life, and plan for it. When it happens, don't go complaining to everyone else about how hard life is – the rest of us are dealing with our own shit and to be honest, we don't really want to hear yours. Behind your back, we just think

you're a moaner. Social media isn't a moaning platform – lighten up, don't wash your dirty laundry in public

- Relax, often, play with your spouse, play with your kids, chill out and be calm
- Get a massage, make it a monthly treat. Take a yoga class whenever you have time, make it every week if you can
- Walk more often, allow time, leave the car at home and walk to the shop or to school
- Walk with your kids, engage them in conversation. Walk with your partner, hold hands, listen to the birds, talk, take time to observe things
- Pray – I have no opinion of your faith, I just know that research shows that people who follow a faith, any faith, live longer
- Make no judgement of others for their faith – it's their business, not yours
- Whatever your faith is, follow it, practice it, celebrate it
- Develop a daily habit of meditation. There's an old saying (and oh boy, this applies to me more than I care to admit) that says "If you can't find 20 minutes a day to meditate, then you need to find an hour a day to meditate." And I think that's probably very true

Time to chill

Stress is a hugely important factor in our understanding of what drives obesity and ill health in our society. It's a major contributing factor in rising rates of obesity, particularly what we call central obesity, which is stored body fat, particularly visceral fat, in your midsection. In short, being stressed out all the time is making you fat.

It's also contributing to type-2 diabetes, metabolic syndrome, high blood pressure, heart disease, stroke, acid reflux, certain autoimmune conditions, IBS, poor bowel function, poor immune function and in some studies it's linked to certain cancers.

Beyond all those long-term effects, in the immediate short term, lifestyle stress is one of the main reasons why people give up on their 'diets' and health efforts and resort to drinking more alcohol than they should and making poor food choices. Think about it, you just can't be super focused on healthy living while you're stressed to hell, buried in debt, and your love life's in the crapper – right? When you are having 'the day from hell' it's highly unlikely that you are going to be super focused on that crunchy organic salad. For most people, nothing drives them to ordering pizza and opening a bottle of wine more than a shitty day at work and an argument with their spouse!

"Low-level, constant lifestyle stress is a major health hazard. Chill out, before you peg out. Value good health over money and possessions – there is no sense in being the richest man in the graveyard."

Summary

- Chronic stress is a contributing causal factor in almost every major chronic lifestyle disease in our society
- Stress causes ill health by interfering with healthy natural hormone function
- It's all about the HPA-axis not working properly (frighteningly technical stuff, best not to ask...and that saves me trying to pretend I understand it!!)
- Over time, this can contribute to obesity, poor immune function, premature ageing and increased risk of life-threatening chronic degenerative disease
- Fight or flight, and rest and digest – your two primary hormonal states: you can't do both at once

- Get a job you enjoy, stop over-spending, borrow less, slow down and smell the roses
- The best ways to combat stress are to get more sleep, take regular exercise, learn to meditate and take more time out to relax
- Love, laugh, smile and pray
- Get more sleep, more sex, more laughter, more smiling. What's not to love about that?

Core Principle 11

There are so many benefits to spending time outside in natural environments that this absolutely needed to be a Core Principle all on its own; it's as important as the food we eat and good hydration. You may think that sounds like an exaggeration, but it's really not. Just think about how many aspects of our lives have changed just in the last 200 to 300 years, really since the Industrial Revolution. Up until about 300 years ago, something like 75% of adult humans worked in agriculture – basically outside all day, in nature, on the land, getting sunshine, fresh air and exercise, working on the land to produce food.

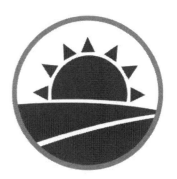

It's only been in historically very recent times that we have shifted to a predominantly indoor, seated, lifestyle. We have never before in millions of years of evolution, had such low exposure to natural sunlight, and been so sedentary. A friend of mine is a GP (MD, for my American readers), and he told me that the three most common complaints he has heard from patients over the last 15 years have been chest infections, depression and low back pain.

Considering everything you have read in this book so far; can you see some possible links here:

- Chest infections: could be because of sub-standard immune function
- Depression: could be caused by or exacerbated by a lack of sunlight and low vitamin D levels[1]
- Low back pain: one major cause is too much sitting down and a lack of physical exercise

---

[1] Anglin, R.E., Samaan, Z., et al (2013). Vitamin D deficiency and depression in adults: systematic review and meta-analysis. *The British Journal of Psychiatry, 202,* 100-7. doi: 10.1192/bjp.bp.111.106666

Can you see how the prevalence of these common health complaints is addressable with some of the simple healthy living advice in this book? Committing to spend more time outside in natural environments, as you will learn in this chapter, can address all those issues and more. *Those are some of the most prevalent health complaints across the nation* – Core Principle 11 is a big part of how the healthy *Mother Nature's Diet* lifestyle addresses those most common problems.

Apart from the direct advantages of spending time in nature, especially around trees, all of which we will get to in a minute, there is also the added bonus that living by this Core Principle will help you to live by several of the others too.

- Core Principle 5 – getting plenty of fresh air. Setting aside time out in nature will help you with that
- Core Principle 9 – regular varied exercise, especially lots of walking, natural movement. Yep, taking time out in nature will help you there too
- Core Principle 10 – reducing stress. Without any doubt, one of the most effective ways to reduce stress is to take time out in nature, to go for long Sunday walks, on the hills, cliff tops, beaches, beside a river, in the woods. Time in beautiful natural places is time away from TV and smartphone screens and time de-stressing
- Core Principle 10 – get more quality sleep. Time spent playing and hiking in nature will definitely aid good healthy sleep at night
- If you spend time outside every day tending your home vegetable garden, then you are living Core Principle 11 while helping to live by Core Principle 7, 8 and 9 at the same time. It's a win:win

Why is time in nature so beneficial?

First, there are practical, physiological and psychological benefits to spending time outside in nature, around trees and in fresh country air:

- Spending time around trees has been shown to have an appreciable positive effect on **asthma** and other diseases. Trees suck up carbon dioxide and put out oxygen, so they help to **reduce air pollution**. Studies show that spending time walking among trees every day has delivered improvements to asthma, heart disease, cancer and stroke recovery

- Improved mental health.[2] Studies show better moods[3], positive stress reduction[4], and reduced depression[5]. One study showed just 90 minutes daily walking in nature showed an appreciable effect on risk factors for depression[6]. How much better would it be to treat depression with a daily walk in the woods, rather than a lifetime of medication? Just get a dog[7] and go out every day, and you'll get endless love from 'man's best friend' too – a double whammy cure for depression without the side effects of medications, or the cost to the NHS

- An aside: at this point, you may be wondering why I filled half this page with scientific references!! I promised a book that was "easy to read" and not too buried in technical details and heavy weight science... Yep, but I am labouring this point, because this is one of the places where the worlds of science and 'woo' are most likely to clash in the middle. I added all these references here just in case anyone thinks "go out walking among the trees" sounds a bit too much like "tree hugging madness". It's not. It's serious, it's good for you, it

---

[2] Harvard Medical School: *Sour mood getting you down? Get back to nature.* (2018, July). Retrieved https://www.health.harvard.edu/mind-and-mood/sour-mood-getting-you-down-get-back-to-nature

[3] *Doctors Explain How Hiking Actually Changes Our Brains.* (2016, April 08). Retrieved from https://www.collective-evolution.com/2016/04/08/doctors-explain-how-hiking-actually-changes-our-brains/

[4] The Atlantic: *How Walking in Nature Prevents Depression.* (2015, June 30). Retrieved from https://www.theatlantic.com/health/archive/2015/06/how-walking-in-nature-prevents-depression/397172/

[5] Scientific American: *Regular Walking Can Help Ease Depression.* (2015, from *American Journal of Preventive Medicine*). Retrieved from https://www.scientificamerican.com/article/regular-walking-can-help-ease-depression/

[6] Bratman, G., et al. (2015). Nature experience reduces rumination and subgenual prefrontal cortex activation. *PNAS* July 14, 2015 112 (28) 8567-8572. https://doi.org/10.1073/pnas.1510459112

[7] National Alliance on Mental Illness: *How Dogs Can Help With Depression.* (2018, Feb 02). Retrieved from https://www.nami.org/Blogs/NAMI-Blog/February-2018/How-Dogs-Can-Help-with-Depression

works. I am not one of those new-age anti-science types, but I do believe that sometimes we humans 'over engineer' solutions to our problems, often problems that are man-made in the first place. For the last hundred years humans have been migrating en masse from rural living to urban living. Two thirds of the human race now live in big towns and cities, and the trend continues. As chronic disease increases, mental health issues certainly seem more prominent than ever, and as our atmosphere suffocates in carbon dioxide - we woefully undervalue trees. Trees are self-growing 'machines' that suck carbon dioxide out of the atmosphere and product oxygen, while locking carbon away in their trunks and underground for decades to come. At the same time as cleaning the air we breathe, just hanging out walking in woodlands can be as effective as taking anti-depressant medications. Don't write Core Principle 11 off as 'woo' because it isn't. You don't have to hug the freakin' trees, just spend time around them, and plant one in your garden if you have some space. Beneficial, proven, it's in the science people...no tin-foil hat bullshit here, just common-sense healthy living

- According to the World Health Organisation, seven million people die prematurely every year because of air pollution[8]. Research suggests that worldwide air pollution is killing more people than smoking[9]. Trees reduce air pollution. Trees soak up air pollutants and provide us with clean air, trees in towns and cities are providing valuable cleaning services and making people healthier

- **Trees make oxygen.** We breathe oxygen. Please don't write this off as insignificant, trees are literally fundamentally important to human life. Oxygen is our most vital nutrient, remember, we die if we go much more than three minutes without it. Oxygen is kind-of a big deal. Trees make our oxygen, all of it

- That's a clue, I think, that trees are pretty important, and we might want to spend more time around them. Maybe I am just some sort of

---

[8] WHO: *7 million premature deaths annually linked to air pollution.* (2014, March 25). Retrieved from
https://www.who.int/mediacentre/news/releases/2014/air-pollution/en/
[9] WE Forum: *Air pollution killing more people than smoking, say scientists.* (2019, March 13). Retrieved from
https://www.weforum.org/agenda/2019/03/air-pollution-killing-more-people-than-smoking-say-scientists

ageing hippie, but I think we have this incredible, beautiful, synergistic relationship with trees. We breathe out what they breath in, they breathe out what we breathe in. Isn't that some kind of beautiful relationship, deserving of mutual respect and appreciation? Yet, we're running around the planet chopping them all down. In broad terms, as the human population **increases**, thanks to our stupidity and greed, the 'tree population' **decreases**. I often wonder: what are we going to do when we chop the last one down? Where will the oxygen come from then? It's very worrying. When there are no trees left, then there will be no people, no 'us'

- Trees promote healing [10]. A 1970s study showed that patients recovering from surgery in hospital, healed faster if they had a view of trees, compared with a view of other buildings. Just looking at trees helped people heal – for real
- Improved cognitive function. Studies have shown that trees help people with clearer thinking, more creative thinking and better problem solving. Kids showed improved cognitive function and got better grades when trees were present in school play grounds[11]
- We should walk on hills from time to time. Psychologists have shown that climbing a hill or mountain and looking down on the land below helps us to feel good. We benefit from feeling like 'the king of the castle' when we look down on land below us, this has appreciable psychological benefits
- Personally, I'm rather obsessed with mountains, so I strongly recommend that everyone tries it sometime - go climb a mountain, come do it with us at *Mother Nature's Diet*, we run several trips every year! Check for the next Mountain Retreat at mothernaturesdiet.com and I'll see you out on the hills!
- Apart from anything else – it's all great exercise!

Quite a lot of people come to *Mother Nature's Diet* overweight and out of shape, and they have not exercised for years, so they are out of condition and not fit and strong enough to start lifting heavy weights or running 10k races. These people tend to start their journey back to regular exercise by initiating

---

[10] Science Daily: *The healing effects of forests.* (2010, July 26). Retrieved from https://www.sciencedaily.com/releases/2010/07/100723161221.htm
[11] More: https://www.phsgreenleaf.co.uk/the-benefits-of-plants-in-schools-and-educational-facilities/

a **daily walking habit**. It's amazing how many people quickly grow to *love and cherish* their daily walk as their most sacred time of the day.

Often that daily walk happens at 5:30am or 6am, perhaps with the family dog, over hills and fields and along quiet country lanes. People take this time to meditate or cogitate on life, and they report back to us that this is their favourite time of the day. Some people develop this habit of walking two, three or four miles every morning, all year (me included 15 to 20 miles per week), whatever the weather, and it becomes the cornerstone of their weight loss efforts and road to improved personal fitness. Don't underestimate the value of taking time out to walk in nature.

Beyond these clear, practical reasons, I believe we must spend time outdoors just because it is so *very nourishing for the soul*.

A basic human right

It would be so easy to think that Core Principle 11 is "the least important one" but that would absolutely not be true. For years I worried that people would not understand how important Core Principle 11 is. Now I realise, it's not that people don't take Core Principle 11 seriously, they do understand it; the real challenge is they **just don't make the time** to actually do it. I'm even *including myself* in there. I make every effort to live the MND way to the letter, but personally my two biggest challenges meeting the MND lifestyle are consistently **getting enough sleep**, and consistently taking enough **time off work**, away from my laptop, to spend time out in nature.

We humans may be the most evolved species on the planet, but we are still an animal like all the others, and we still come from an evolutionary line that spent millions and millions of years living in and on the Earth like all animals do. It's only been in very recent times, in terms of our evolutionary jounrney, that we started 'separating' ourselves from the Earth and the environment, physically, with 'barriers' between us and the natural world – by barriers I mean clothes, shoes, socks, air conditioning, double-glazing, concrete floors, brick walls, steel boxes (our cars), sunglasses, hats and so on.

Now, of course, I am not suggesting you run around in public naked in the middle of winter, but what we need to recognise is that we are insulating ourselves from many beneficial elements of the natural world, such as the vitamin D producing benefits of sunlight on our skin, the gut-healthy world of microbes and bacteria (that live in the soil, literally in the Earth), and the soul-enriching, freedom-enhancing joy of spending time in wild, natural places.

Yet again, these subjects could all be the topics of entire books on their own, and there simply is not space to do all this justice here. The gut microbiome is a relatively new and rapidly expanding area of science that we are learning more about every year. We are increasingly learning that many families of bacteria are our friends, they help our digestion and immune system in previously unknown ways. Healthy unpolluted soil is teeming with literally billions of bacteria in every teaspoon, it does us good to sit and picnic down on the ground, to walk barefoot on the Earth, and to get those microbes on our skin, and on our hands.[12]

Researchers have taken under-privileged inner-city kids from deprived areas out to the countryside for experience days on working farms, and seen these kids light up with creativity, enthusiasm and cognitive abilities. Studies have shown that just digging your bare hands into fresh healthy soil is both pleasurable and instantly improves cognition.

We all know how it feels good to walk barefoot on a soft sandy beach, but it also feels good to walk barefoot on wet grass, or on damp soft soils. It feels wonderful walking on wet mud, on the hills, in muddy puddles in the rain, you should try it some time. Folks are out there buying sugary confectionery or online shopping or online gambling as 'cheap thrill' therapy to make them happy. Instead, go walking barefoot in a muddy field when it's raining - it's free, and good for you, try it. I'm serious, it feels fabulous, it makes you feel so alive. Take your kids out to walk barefoot in wet mud, it's wonderful good fun.

Spending time around plants and touching soil has been shown to boost immune system function, healthy soil is full of minerals, it's not 'dirt', it's not *dirty*...it's healthy, it's where most of our food comes from. Fertile topsoil is the very crucible of life on Earth, down in the soil is where all our food grows, it's the bed of nutrients that keep us alive. Don't be afraid of soil, it's teeming with life, all far too small for us to see, but all an essential part of the food cycle on Earth. Without soil, all life on the land would soon cease to exist.[13]

Please do not under-estimate the importance of spending time outside in natural places. Walk in the woods, climb a few hills, stroll barefoot on the

---

[12] Nurminen, N., et al. (2018). Nature-derived microbiota exposure as a novel immunomodulatory approach. *Future Medicine*, Vol. 13, No. 7. https://doi.org/10.2217/fmb-2017-0286
[13] *What Are Microbes: The Benefits Of Microbes In Soil.* (Updated 2018). Retrieved from https://www.gardeningknowhow.com/garden-how-to/soil-fertilizers/what-are-microbes-in-soil.htm

beach. This is important stuff, it really is fundamentally good for you in so many ways.

> If you live in a city, try to spend time in the countryside whenever possible, take **weekend trips** out for long walks. If you work in the city, can you go walk in a park in your lunch break?
>
> It stands to reason that you will be breathing in cleaner air walking in the fields and woodlands, than in the middle of the city, where cars are all around. Find parks. Find trees.
>
> Along with heart disease and cancer, lung diseases are the other big player in the top three killers in our society. Look after your lungs, find trees and green spaces to go for walks, jogging or bike rides.

Sunshine and vitamin D

Oh dear, sunshine is another of those widely misunderstood and hotly contested topics in the world of health, fitness and nutrition. I fear that throughout this book I have told you too many times that such-and-such is the most argued about topic in nutrition...is it carbs, is it calories, now is it whether or not sunshine causes skin cancer?! More glorious confusion! Let's get to the facts.

Vitamin D is an essential micronutrient, like the other vitamins, and we would be in big trouble without any. In fact, vitamin D is one of the most important vitamins, and once inside our bodies, vitamin D actually converts into a steroid hormone that is massively important for many bodily functions. The many roles of this hormone include over 650 metabolic processes, and it plays a vital role in regulating many of our genes, something close to almost 5% of all the protein-encoding genes in the human body.[14]

If that doesn't mean much to you, don't worry, just know that vitamin D is very important and helps with a gazillion things from helping us to have

---

[14] Wacker, M., & Holick, M. F. (2013). Sunlight and Vitamin D. A global perspective for health. *Dermato-endocrinology.* 2013 Jan 1; 5(1): 51–108. doi: 10.4161/derm.24494

strong bones, to helping our metabolism to work properly; from helping with growth and development, to helping protect us from cancer.

The best source of vitamin D is, of course, sunlight. When you get sunlight on large areas of your skin, it will convert cholesterol into vitamin D inside your body. (Ummm, interesting, another valuable role for cholesterol...such an important substance!)[15] Sunlight is by far the best source of vitamin D.

There are some good ways to get vitamin D in your diet, yes, such as eating oily fish and free-range eggs, but exposing your skin to the sunshine, during the warmest times of the year (here in the UK), is definitely your best option.

To give you an idea of how important sunlight is; ten minutes with your shirt off, or in a sleeveless top, crop-top or vest, exposing large amounts of your skin to the sun, in the sunny half of the year in the middle of the day, when the sun's nice and warm, ten minutes will give you the same amount of vitamin D as eating three-and-a-half pounds of fresh salmon. So, do you want half-a-pound of salmon for breakfast every day, or take ten or fifteen minutes in your lunch break to lay in the sun in the park, eating your organic salad, catching rays?

That last sentence, that just ticked off seven of the 12 Core Principles in one go. Did you spot that? Can you see how easy that was to put together all these Core Principles...?

- Core Principle 1 (swap the sandwich for a salad)
- Core Principle 5 (go out at lunchtime and get some fresh air)
- Core Principle 7 (salad, it's plants and animals)
- Core Principle 8 (I said the salad was organic)
- Core Principle 9 (exercise, walk to the park in your lunch break)
- Core Principle 10 (reduce stress, take a break, go to the park)
- Core Principle 11 (time among the trees, lying in the grass, getting some sunshine)

We're clear that vitamin D is good for you, and the best way to get vitamin D is to get as much sun as you can during the warm half of the year, and eat a good diet that includes oily fish. That leaves two questions:

---

[15] Harvard Medical School: *Vitamin D and your health: Breaking old rules, raising new hopes.* (2007, Feb). Retrieved from https://www.health.harvard.edu/newsletter_article/vitamin-d-and-your-health-breaking-old-rules-raising-new-hopes

1. What do we do for vitamin D during winter?
2. Doesn't sun exposure cause skin cancer?

Generally, I am not a big fan of the supplement industry, because the truth is that there is no substantial scientific evidence [16] to show that taking supplements works. Some studies even seem to show[17] that taking broad range multi-vitamin and mineral supplements in predominantly healthy people, actually can do more harm than good. But then I remember one of the core lessons of this book: **one size does not fit all.**

There can be many reasons to take a supplement, and many reasons or examples where supplements may prove beneficial; and there can be many reasons and examples why supplements failed to provide any benefits. Let's not side-track off into all that now. Let's just understand this:

- Vitamins and minerals are good for us
- They are best obtained from a **whole-foods based diet**
- They are best absorbed and utilised **from whole foods**, because in whole foods they are 'packaged' in balance, all in the right quantities in relation to each other, to aid optimal assimilation by our body
- Packaged in whole foods, these nutrients are also bound up with fibre, starch, fat and protein, which slows the speed with which they are delivered to our digestive system, allowing us time to absorb them in the right quantity at the right time
- Delivered as a pill, all of the above factors are absent, and so it seems, are many of the benefits of the vitamins and minerals
- If you have ever taken a large so-called 'mega-dose' vitamin B-group supplement, you may have noticed that you pee turns orange an hour later. That is your body pee'ing out most of that expensive vitamin B2 you just swallowed, simply because your body cannot

---

[16] Emerging Data Continue to Find Lack of Benefit for Vitamin-Mineral Supplement Use. (2014, Feb 5). *JAMA*. 2014;311(5):454-455. doi:10.1001/jama.2013.285786

[17] Bjelakovic G, Nikolova D, Gluud LL, Simonetti RG, Gluud C. (2012) Antioxidant supplements for prevention of mortality in healthy participants and patients with various diseases. *Cochrane Database of Systematic Reviews* 2012, Issue 3. Art. No.: CD007176. DOI: 10.1002/14651858.CD007176.pub2

utilise so much of it delivered in such a condensed form, all at once. That's a total waste of your money

For these reasons, I generally advise healthy people not to bother taking broad-range vitamin and mineral supplements, and those 'tonic' drinks, and instead just to eat a nutrient-dense whole-foods diet, the way I have explained throughout this book, to meet all your micronutrient needs.

However, that's for broadly healthy people. By contrast, there may be plenty of occasions when an unhealthy person needs a supplement, to help recover from an illness or surgery, to help correct an imbalance, or to supplement a long-term dietary weakness (such as a vegan taking B12.) Clearly, one size does not fit all.

With all that said, I do not push, sell or recommend supplements for anyone, but I do know that approximately 75% of Brits are estimated to be somewhat vitamin D deficient, and so I would recommend that you take a test and consider a supplement for the winter half of the year. You can order a simple home test online, it'll probably cost about £30 or £40, and they send you a little kit in the post. You take a finger prick, squeeze a few drops of blood into a test tube, and send it back for testing. In a few days, you'll know the result. If you are vitamin D deficient, maybe you should take a modest-strength supplement daily for six months of the year.

But don't just take the pills – get tested first, to see if you really need them. Now, that has answered the first question. The second question was about skin cancer risks.

Does sun exposure cause skin cancer?

The short answer is 'no', regular responsible sun exposure does not cause skin cancer, whereas the long-term health issues associated with chronic vitamin D deficiency, and chronic lack of sun exposure, causes more health problems, serious ones, that could be avoided. The key word in all of this is **'responsible'**.

The science shows that sun exposure is beneficial in many ways. A lack of vitamin D, and a lack of sun exposure in general, appears to contribute to heart disease, various cancers, diabetes, Alzheimer's disease, macular degeneration, dementia and multiple sclerosis,[18] many of which are more serious life-threatening conditions than skin cancer. If found early, skin cancers can be highly treatable[19], and many are cured quite easily.

Overall, the science suggests (and this stuff comes up every few years – 2003, 2006, 2008, 2013, 2016, it's quite regular) that the benefits of sun exposure far outweigh any increased risk of skin cancer[20]. But again, one size does not fit all, and some people may want to be more careful than others, perhaps if there is a strong family history of skin cancer.

Responsible

Above all, responsible is the watch-word in all of this. What does that mean? You can live the *Mother Nature's Diet* way, which means you spend time outside every day of your life, maybe you walk your dog every morning, you enjoy playing an outdoor sport once per week, you go out jogging or riding your bike once or twice per week, you stroll in the park during your lunch break, and you do some gardening and enjoy long countryside walks with a loved one or with your kids on the weekend.

Whenever it's nice, you get some skin on show, wear a vest or sleeveless top, or take your shirt off. You spend lots of time outside in summer, working on your garden, enjoying long bike rides and a sunny annual holiday. You love to sunbathe, you make the most of it during the short summer we get here in the UK, and you generally get a decent tan every summer. When it gets too much and you feel yourself going pink, you slip on a top or move in to the shade. That's what year-round **responsible sun exposure** looks like.

Conversely, what is not responsible?

---

[18] Hoel, D. G., Berwick, M., de Gruijl, F. R., & Holick, M. F. (2016). The risks and benefits of sun exposure 2016. *Dermato-endocrinology,* 8(1), e1248325. doi:10.1080/19381980.2016.1248325

[19] Skin Cancer Foundation: *If You Can Spot It You Can Stop It.* See: https://www.skincancer.org/skin-cancer-information/early-detection/if-you-can-spot-it-you-can-stop-it

[20] Medical News Today: *Sun Exposure Benefits May Outweigh Risks Say Scientists.* (2013, May 8). Retrieved from https://www.medicalnewstoday.com/articles/260247.php

You're one of those pasty white people who has not worn shorts since 1985, your skin is so white that if you took your shirt off outside the trees would have to put sunglasses on because of the glare. You say that you don't sunbathe because "I'm one of those people, I hate it, I just burn really easily" and you never get a tan. You work 14-hours per day in an air-conditioned office, you don't use your garden at home, never wear short sleeves, and never use your annual holiday allowance...until August. Then you get a plane, fly 3000 miles south and suddenly don swimwear and hit the beach for 10 hours straight laying spread-eagle in blistering 35-degree sunshine.

That's dumb. That's **irresponsible sun exposure**. That's going to increase burns, and skin cancer risks.

Can you see the difference between the sensible way to benefit from lots of sun exposure, and the stupid way to burn and hurt yourself?

Disconnect for a day, watch less TV, get offline

Core Principle 11 is all about reconnecting with nature. It's about backing off the man-made structures of the modern world a little, even if it's just one day a week, and taking some time to re-wild yourself a little bit. That's not anti-science, it's not anti-modernism, we're not running around screaming "smash the spinning jenny", it's just an attempt to re-establish some healthy connection with nature.

In my opinion, a lot of people watch *far too much TV these days*. Try to cut back, maybe plan yourself one day a week where you don't watch any. Take some time offline. Perhaps lying in bed at midnight with your tablet or smartphone, logged in to your favourite social media channel reading other people's arguments and opinions about politics and religion isn't the most brilliant way to calm your mind down for a good night's sleep. Instead, disconnect, leave the phone and tablet in another room and read a good book instead.

Tree hugger

Spending time in natural environments has been shown to improve vitality, mood and libido. Get out of the air conditioning, get away from the TV, turn off the Internet connection, put the smartphone away and take a break outside. If you live in a city, book a few weekends away each year, get out to the countryside and go camping, try to find somewhere with no mobile phone coverage, force yourself to detox from the digital world.

Make no excuses, get out there and get connected with Mother Nature. It's good for you in every imaginable way! You don't have to become an unshaven long-haired tree hugger (unless you want to, that's fine!), just make some time every week to spend outside in beautiful, natural places. It can be so uplifting for your soul.

In my life I have never met anyone who spent time out in the countryside, wandering along cliff tops in the sunshine, listening to the birds and catching a tan, who said at the end "Oh yuk that was awful, I feel so dirty and stressed...I can't wait to get back in to the city to feel clean and fresh again." Never!! Time in nature is hugely beneficial and massively important, you must make it happen.

Spend time in nature

Go out on the weekends, go for a walk in the woods, hold the hand of someone you love, take the dog, walk on the hills, walk along that clifftop path, look at the ocean, walk on the beach, just do it. There are extensive benefits to spending time outside in natural environments: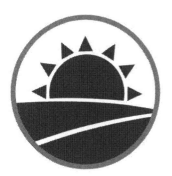

- Trees reduce air pollution
- Trees make oxygen
- Time around trees shown to help reduce symptoms of asthma
- Helps in treatment of depression, dementia, cancer and heart disease
- Aids recovery from stroke, asthma and surgery
- Helps you to live by Core Principles 5, 7, 8, 9 and 10
- Improves cognitive function and mental well-being
- Studies – and sheer common sense – show that spending time outside reduces stress and improves quality of sleep
- This is not tree-hugger 'woo-woo' quack science, this is real, time in forests, around tress, and in natural environments, is good for us physically, and good for our mental wellbeing, in many proven and measurable ways

196

- It just makes us feel good – isn't that, alone, enough?
- More oxygen for your body (Core Principle 5)
- Enjoyable beneficial exercise (move naturally, remember?)
- Aids clear and creative thinking
- Connect with the earth for beneficial bacteria and microbes, it's good for your gut function and your immune system
- Get plenty of sunshine, for vitamin D among other benefits, and remember that sun exposure is far more effective than diet for vitamin D
- Vitamin D as a supplement is a back-up plan at best – it's not the optimal solution
- Get lots of sun exposure. **Responsible sun exposure**
- Watch less TV, cut back on social media, disconnect for a day, a regular digital detox is good for you
- Gardening counts! Gardening is great time outside connecting with nature. Start growing a few veg in a spare flower bed at home, it will help you with Core Principle 8 as well as Core Principle 11, you have nothing to lose!

Everyone enjoys time outside in the beauty and calm of Mother Nature. Sunset walks, family picnics, meadows of wild flowers. It's good for your mind, body and soul.

You can use this page for your own notes.

Core Principle 12

Some people will find it difficult implementing Core Principles 1 through 11 into their lives. For some people, ditching bread will be hard; for some people getting off their sugar addiction will be hard; for some people quitting or cutting right back on alcohol will be the biggest challenge. Some people will find it pretty easy making these changes, and other folks may find it all quite tough. That's just how it is, we all face our own demons, our own emotional issues, our own life circumstances, and that makes a weight loss journey or a health program different for each and every one of us.

Go easy on yourself. *Mother Nature's Diet* is a healthy lifestyle.

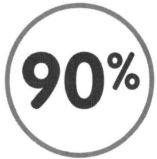

- It's not a fad
- It's not torture
- It's not punishment
- It's not meant to be hard
- And it's most definitely not a 'bandwagon'!

Core Principle 12 is your safety net, your 'pressure release valve' to make the whole *Mother Nature's Diet* lifestyle easier, more manageable and completely long-term sustainable.

Core Principle 10 was all about reducing stress, so the last thing we want is to try to be a diet perfectionist and get stressed out about our food. If you are out to a business lunch and you look at the menu and it doesn't state that the beef is grass-fed, no drama. You don't need to ask the client if you can go to a different restaurant, no sweat if the vegetables aren't organic. Just pick something from the menu that fits 'plants and animals' and make do with that.

You see, that's Core Principle 12 at work. It's there to say "get it right 90% of the time, then chill out over the last 10%, no drama." It's there to make life easier, and to make this healthy lifestyle realistic, achievable and sustainable for the long term.

If you go to friends for a meal, and they serve pasta, just relax, eat it, this one time it won't hurt. But politely decline the dessert, because two wrongs don't make a right! This is the idea of Core Principle 12. It's there to make life easier, so you don't become one of those boring, fussy food-nerds who no one wants to hang out with, and to stop you feeling stressed about your food choices. Core Principle 12 allows you to get it right 90% of the time, and relax about the last 10%.

What does Core Principle 12 allow?

- If you can't afford organic all the time, then buy organic for the so-called 'dirty dozen' which use the most pesticides (includes apples, peaches, spinach, tomatoes and bell peppers – you can look up 'the dirty dozen' online any time, it changes every year, as farmer's use of pesticides change with the seasons)[1]
- Buy organic for the things where you eat the outer skin, like spinach and broccoli, but save your money on grapefruits, pineapples and melon
- If moderate alcohol consumption suits you better than teetotal, then that's OK
- If you want to have an ice cream while you're on the beach with your kids on summer holiday, then chill out and enjoy. Just make sure it's only a couple of ice creams per holiday, not a couple every day!
- If you are in a restaurant and can't find pasture-fed meat, no stress this one time, just order what they have
- If you dine out and eat dessert, don't beat yourself up about it, just don't do it every day. If you dine in restaurants once a month, then dessert once in a while won't hurt, but if you dine in restaurants three or four times per week, you need to exercise more restraint

Can you see how this works? It's just common sense - no crazy, no drama.

---

[1] Changes annually. See EWG website at
https://www.ewg.org/foodnews/dirty-dozen.php

Our goal is progress, not perfection.

It's about being sensible, taking the drama out of healthy living, making it sustainable. We all accept that in our modern world, foods made from grains, starchy carbs and sugar are everywhere, and sometimes we get caught away from home and in need of food and we have to make the best choice we can from what is available. Trying to religiously avoid sugar and grains and processed foods 100% of the time is virtually impossible.

But if that situation arises, and you just have to buy something, and you reject the white bread sandwiches and settle on a chicken salad in a multi-seed tortilla wrap, then you haven't done too badly at all. You can tick that off under Core Principle 12 and feel pleased with yourself that you made the best choice available. At least you didn't default to a box of sugary donuts!

The goal is to **do the best we can** with what is available. It's about making progress, rather than seeking outright perfection. This journey to supreme good health; **it's a marathon, not a sprint.** What you do *most* of the time will define your results, not what you do occasionally.

What you do most of the time will define your results, not what you do occasionally.

What does Core Principle 12 not allow?

- It's not an excuse to binge!
- MND is not a fad diet! You can't just do this for 30 days, drop three dress sizes and then go back to a diet of cake and daytime TV, that shit doesn't work! This is a lifestyle, it's about making permanent change, it's about living smarter, for life

- Eating fish and veggies from Monday to Friday, then blowing out all weekend on junk food and heavy drinking is not "enjoying your 10%" and that's not what this is about
- It's not a 'cheat day' or an 'allowance' of 'sin points'
- It's not an excuse to get blind drunk once per week and pig out on junk food

Mother Nature's Diet is a commitment to yourself, to be the best version of you that you can be, **it's a long-term healthy lifestyle**. It's not rocket science, it's all pretty simple stuff. Many people are overweight, out of shape, tired all the time and suffering a range of minor chronic health conditions. The advice in the 12 Core Principles can help with all that, **but you have to do this stuff**, you have to make the choices, exercise some self-control, make better decisions. It's about personal responsibility. You may recall...**you have a choice.**

You are going to have to change. If you keep doing what you've been doing, you'll keep getting what you've been getting.

Core Principle 12 is here as a 'safety valve' to help you manage that change without feeling like you are living under some strict, crazy, fad diet regime. Ultimately, how much you apply this stuff, how 'strict' you are, will largely determine the speed with which you get the results. Some people go for it 100%, they live the Core Principles 1 through 11 to the letter, and they get great results, fast. Others push Core Principle 12 to the limit and live the MND way at about 70/30...and they still get beneficial results, but much slower, the changes take much longer, but that suits some people, so that's OK by me.

How it works for you...is entirely up to you. In this life, you get out what you put in. Your results are up to you. That's your personal responsibility.

It is always worth remembering that what we do *occasionally* has comparatively little impact on our results, it's what we do *habitually* that really defines us. It's not what you do once in a while that counts, it's what you do 90% of the time that determines your results.

Our habits define us.
Consistency is king.

You will learn more about the importance of consistency in the next chapter, as we begin to pull everything together and lay out a plan for forward progress.

If you're making the right choices 90 or 95% of the time, you're going to be getting the improved health outcomes that you want. You're going to have the energy levels you want, the health you want, the vitality you want. Your ability to lose weight, resist ill health, all those things you want, they come when you stick to the plan, when you give up fad diet behaviour and adopt a permanent healthy lifestyle for the long term.

Don't follow the herd

We know that three quarters of the population are making the wrong choices.

- 73% of British adults don't eat their 5-a-day
- Approximately 70% to 75% of Brits are somewhat vitamin D deficient
- 60% of UK adult men and 70% of UK adult women do not take the government's advice for the recommended minimum amount of exercise in a week – and that's a bar that is set pretty low to start with
- 20% of UK adults still smoke
- 72% of Brits do not eat the recommended minimum of two servings of fish per week
- Approximately 99% of food sold in the UK is not organic

The sad truth is that most people are making pretty poor choices. These numbers are for the UK, but if I were to run similar data for the United States, or for many countries across Europe, we would find a similar pattern.

Sometimes that may be that people don't care, they are lazy, or they are more interested in saving money...but I actually think that in a lot of cases, it's because those people *don't know* what you know, **now that you have read this book.**

You have a choice. Most people just don't understand that.

Personally, if I'm completely hand-on-heart honest, I live about 97/3. So, about 97% of calories that ever pass my lips meet Core Principles 1 through to 11. Then 3% is tucked under my Core Principle 12. It's a few squares of organic dark chocolate (85%, yummy, very little sugar), or it's an ice cream on summer holidays, or it's a pizza on my kids' birthday.

I would encourage you to spend 90-95% of your time making the right choices, especially as you get older. If you're 26, you can get away with murder and you have plenty of time on your side to sort things out. But if you're 56, your body will be less forgiving, your metabolism and hormones less forgiving. If you're out of shape at 56, then you have some serious work to do to get things back on track. Core Principle 12 might mean 75/25 or 80/20 for folks in their 30s, but it might mean 95/05 for folks in their 50s and 60s. Again, one size does not fit all.

Meanwhile, back in the real world...

Time for a quick reality check. That's how I wrote CP 12, everything over the last few pages, that's what it is meant to mean – don't sweat the detail, don't stress over the minutiae, don't alienate yourself from friends and family by being the boring nerd who takes on some annoying air of superiority over your diet (that person just annoys everyone and comes across as arrogant, and everyone thinks he or she is a total dick. Take note my haughty 'vegan-superior' friends.)

But in reality, that's actually not how most people interpret and live by Core Principle 12! For eight years now, I have been promoting the 12 Core Principles, and I find most people actually live CP 12 as "I live by the MND way 90% of the time, and then I do and eat what the hell I like the other 10% of the time!"

You know what, **that's OK, if you want to do that, then do that, it's OK by me.** If you are getting things right 90% of the time, then you are doing better than 75% to 80% of other people in this country, and I am proud of you.

Many adapt Core Principle 12 to 80/20 or even 70/30. I have people come up to me and tell me they are 50/50 and they smile and say "It's the healthiest diet I have ever eaten in my life!" They are proud of that 50/50, because it's a huge improvement over the four fizzy cola drinks per day, the microwave dinners they were eating before, and the beers every evening. You have to do what is best for you. The goal is progress, not perfection.

Summary – Core Principle 12

Core Principle 12 is all about making the *Mother Nature's Diet* lifestyle easy, manageable and sustainable in the long term. This book started by explaining that fad diets mostly don't work, because all too often the 'regime' is too strict, the rules are too tough to stick to, and folks fall off the wagon.

So MND includes Core Principle 12 to help you stay on track, it's your safety valve, to release a little pressure and keep you sane.

You have learned:

- Consistency is king!
- Get it all right 90% of the time and you will be doing great
- **The faster you want to get results, the stricter you need to be**
- Chill out, go easy on yourself, if you mess up one day, and you will, then that's OK, it's no big deal, don't berate yourself for it, just crack on and do better the next day

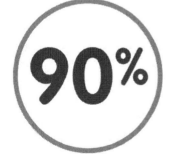

- Our goal is progress, not perfection
- You got this, you can do this
- **It's not an excuse to binge on junk**
- On plan Monday-to-Friday then blow out all weekend is not 90/10!

- Core Principle 12 is not a regular 'cheat day' (you are only cheating yourself!) or a weekly allowance...it is flexibility, that you may use more one month (maybe, December) and less another (maybe, January) but it allows you to live a normal balanced life without becoming a 'food nerd'
- It's not what you do once in a while that counts, it's what you do 90% of the time that determines your results
- Our habits define us
- Did I mention – consistency is king!
- The older you are, the more you need to stick to the rules
- Don't follow the herd
- You have a choice

"What you do __most__ of the time will define your results, not what you do occasionally."

Bringing It All Together

Yippee, well done, you made it, you've got this far, you've made it through the 12 Core Principles – congratulations! Now, for the last few chapters of the book, we'll summarise what we have learned, pull it all together into a plan for your journey forward, and answer some frequently asked questions.

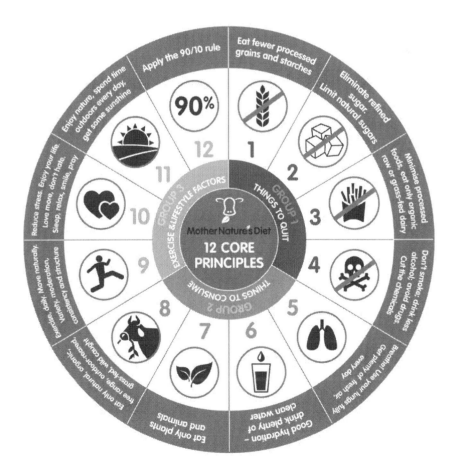

You will have realised that the 12 Core Principles are organised in three clear groups.

- **Group 1** is all about things to take out of your diet. The goal is to stop putting in foods that are not serving you optimally; they may be contributing to weight gain, weakening your immune system, or just not nourishing you very well
- **Group 2** is all about putting things in to your diet to nourish and replace the things we took out in Group 1, to provide you wish optimal function, more energy and the best possible ability to resist the signs of ageing and ill health
- **Group 3** is all about lifestyle factors to support the dietary changes made between Group 1 and 2, and to help you achieve supreme good health through less stress and more sleep and exercise

The three groups work together, obviously. The things we add to our diet in Group 2 replace the things we cut back in Group 1, and Group 3 offers lifestyle support to make it all a little easier – believe me, living without cake and wine and eating more fish and cabbage instead is much easier when you are not stressed out or exhausted with tiredness! Give it some time, and you will learn to love the fish and cabbage, and you won't miss the cake and wine at all! **That really is true!** But it does take some time, so you need to be patient and consistent.

Along the way, it's worth noting:

- Only half of the 12 Core Principles actually have anything to do with food
- There are twice as many Principles about what to stop putting in, as there are telling you what you should actually consume
- Out of 12, only 2 of them actually tell you what food to eat
- **The 12 Core Principles are planned out that way on purpose –** there are clues in that arrangement!
- Most people need to focus *twice as much* on eating less (and eating less of the *wrong* foods) than they do on new recipe ideas and meal planning
- Unlike most diet books that focus almost entirely on food, packing 300 pages with recipes and pictures of food, in reality most people who need to lose weight already seem to be pretty good at the whole eating thing...they need to take their focus off food, stop thinking

about food and eating so much, and refocus their attention on other areas – like exercise, fresh air, time outside, sunshine and so on

- Instead of being 300 pages of recipes and pictures of food, this book is 300 pages of lifestyle advice, loaded with talk of exercise, sleep, water, stress reduction, fresh air, nature and walking. That's all for a reason!!

- Most folks don't need more recipes and more advice on what to eat...they need advice on what to not eat, what to stop putting in, and they need advice on how to exercise and move more, and reduce stress and get more/better sleep

- There are 4 Principles on what to stop eating, 2 on what to eat. There are 4 Core Principles on the benefits of getting outside every day – 5, 9, 10 and 11 all talk about getting outside every day for some natural movement time – that's how important that is, it's as important as getting all the wrong foods out of your diet

- Get off your butt, get on your feet, get outside, in daylight...move naturally, spend more time in natural environments, move more

- Society is awash with mental health problems...and it's only going to get worse as the human population increasingly moves to urbanisation...time outside in nature, access to trees, parks, daylight, sunshine, has never been more important

I hope you can see how the 12 Core Principles are structured in this way, 'weighted' according to the importance of each area. It's all by design. You should treat all 12 with equal importance, they are all meant to be as important as each other.

How we have been through the 12 Core Principles in some detail, I want to remind you of something I wrote back at the start, on Page 35:

"...that's why I often say that the 12 Core Principles of *Mother Nature's Diet* are guidelines, sign posts to help you navigate your way to find the perfect diet for you."

"...Given that *we are all different*, and given that the perfect healthy diet for anyone **is the healthy diet they stick to**, these 12 simple one-liners, in the plainest English possible, make a solid starting foundation for most people. But they are **not** a one-size-fits-all prescription. That's just *not possible*. You need to try these Core Principles out, and find the ones that work for you as an individual."

That is my wish for you, that you will try out the advice in this book, to find the bits that work for you, and tailor the *Mother Nature's Diet* way to suit you perfectly. That might mean a slightly different end-result for everyone, and that's great. One person will enjoy running, one won't. One person will thrive on "low carbs and lots of meat" while another won't. One person will suit mostly plant-based eating, loads of veggies, and one person won't. One person will enjoy lifting weights, and one person won't. Try out the ideas in this book, to find the lifestyle that works best for you.

The 12 Core Principles in summary:

- Cut back on eating so much starchy carbohydrate. Maybe 50 or 60 years ago, when we didn't have two or three cars to every family, and an electrically-powered labour-saving device for almost every household task, maybe then we needed all that extra carbohydrate for energy. But these days, folks don't move as much as they used to, and they don't use their muscles as often, jobs are less manual and more office-based, and in my experience most folks just don't need all those carbs every day. Additionally, the carbs these days are far more refined, it's all added sugar, white bread, white pasta and spaghetti, rice, bagels and so on. Too much sugar, eaten too often, is leading to weight gain and contributing to metabolic syndrome

- Refined sugar – as a society, we eat far too much sweet food. It offers very little nutritional value, cut that stuff right out for weight loss and better health

- Keep processed foods to an absolute minimum. They offer low nutritional value and usually have added sugar. Spend your money on nutrition, not packaging

- Don't smoke. Drink less. Keep your lifetime exposure to man-made chemicals to a minimum (think cosmetics, household chemicals, chemicals at work, pesticides, air pollution)

- Get some clean fresh air – get outside and use your lungs every day

- Drink plenty of fresh clean water, many people mistake thirst for hunger

- Eat fresh whole foods – plants and animals. 95% of your diet should come from vegetables, fish, eggs, meat, organ meats, poultry, fruits, nuts and seeds

- Buy organic. What you save on buying less alcohol and confectionery and cosmetics, you can spend on that top-quality grass-fed meat. Try growing a few of your own veggies at home, it's easy once you get started

- Exercise, aim for something every day, even if it's just a walk. Consistency is king. Go for variety – sometimes puffing and panting, sometimes engaging your muscles, sometimes gentle stretching. Variety and consistency rule. Try a yoga class
- Reduce stress in your life. Sleep more, it's the best antidote to chronic stress. Ensure your bedroom is dark, calm, quiet and cool
- Take a day offline from time to time. Watch less TV. Take time to nourish your soul. Share time with those you love. Have more sex. Learn to meditate. Laugh more often
- Get outside in nature as often as you can. It's good for you in so many ways you don't realise. Get some sunshine – little and often is the best way to go
- Get it all right 90% of the time. Chill out over the last 10%. No drama

That's it. 12 simple steps to living a healthy life, to being the best version of you that you can be. 12 simple ways to maintain a healthy bodyweight, look and feel your best for life, have more energy and do your best to avoid ill health and chronic disease.

Healthy living really boils down to a handful of rather ordinary, common-sense good ideas. Do yourself a favour; avoid the fad diets, stay away from the supplements, superfoods and 'snake oil' solutions, and embrace the *Mother Nature's Diet* healthy lifestyle. No bullshit, just simple, sustainable, effective healthy living.

You can use this page for your own notes.

The Pyramid

This chapter mainly relates to people on a weight loss journey, personal transformation, or a journey from poor health to good. This graphic illustrates the factors that underpin a healthy lifestyle, showing them in *approximate proportions* of how important they are. In *proportion*: that means the wider the segment on the pyramid, the more important the factors. The big things at the bottom of the pyramid are *the most important*, the little things at the top are really just 'the icing on the cake'.

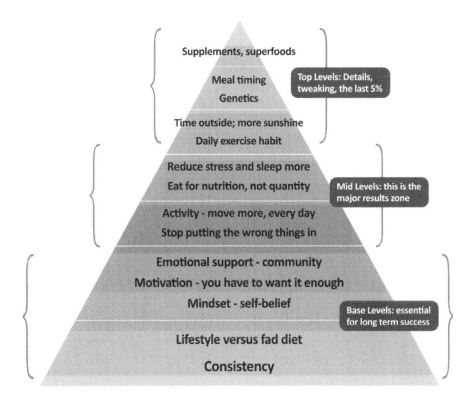

The Pyramid of Success Factors

What is it?

The Pyramid shows factors that are likely to determine your success or failure in changing your lifestyle from one full of unhealthy habits to a healthier way of living. These are factors that will play a vital role in your success or failure in a major weight loss drive.

It's not a ranking of how important 'things' are to your overall health. If it was, breathing air would be at the bottom. Then drinking water. Then sleep. Then food.

How and why is this relevant?

Start at the bottom, then move up. From my experience over the last decade trying to help people to adopt a healthier lifestyle, I find that the factors in the base levels of the pyramid are by far the most important things.

I have never met anyone who blamed their 10, 20 or 30 years of failed yo-yo diets on "well I just don't think I was getting enough sleep" or "my hydration wasn't on point" or "I just didn't use the right ab machine down the gym."

Good sleep is important, you'll die without it. Hydration is important, you'll die without it. Exercise is important in many ways. However, **making mistakes in these areas are rarely why people fail at attempts to lose weight** and change to a healthier lifestyle.

Far more commonly, what I hear is this:

"Every time I try to diet my husband ridicules me and tells me to stop wasting my time because I always fail."

And: *"I always start really well but then after a week or two family and work hassles distract me and before you know it, I'm back to square one."*

And: *"I tried that diet but it doesn't work, it's just impossible to stick to the plan they give you, the powders cost a fortune and counting calories drives me mad!"*

Lack of **consistency**, lack of **support** and **fad diet behaviour** are often the classic 'traps' people fall into. Without these foundation stones in place, changing a couple of decades of habitual behaviour for a better future is incredibly difficult.

Context:
- The 28-Day Plan, coming up in about 15 pages, is 'What to do'
- This whole book is 'Why to do it'
- This Pyramid of Success Factors is what you need in place to underpin your efforts

Let's dig into the layers of The Pyramid and make more sense of the thinking behind each of these factors.

The Base Levels

The Base Levels of the pyramid, the bottom third, are the major foundations to a healthy life, and from my experience I would reluctantly admit that, frankly, in all honesty, without getting these things sorted first, long term success in weight loss and optimum health is unlikely.

These big factors down here in the bottom third of the pyramid are mostly all about how you think, it's all mindset and psychology. If this mindset stuff is off, you're in trouble.

- **Consistency:** it's not what you do once in a while that defines you, it's your habits, your daily practises, that determine your success. No diet or healthy lifestyle plan will work if you don't stick to it. **The perfect diet, is the one you stick to.** Consistency is #1, the most important thing, above all others
- **Lifestyle versus fad diet:** fad diets lead to fad results. The route to being a healthy person is to live a healthy lifestyle
- **Core Principle 12:** it's down here that Core Principle 12 keeps you sane, keeps you on track. You can use Core Principle 12 to adjust the *Mother Nature's Diet* lifestyle to be your perfect diet – *the diet that you stick to*
- **Mindset, self-belief:** if you don't *think* you *can* change, if you don't think you *can* lose weight, if you don't think you *can* stick to a healthy lifestyle, then you probably won't. As Henry Ford famously said *"Whether you think you can, or you think you can't, you're right."* You have to believe in what you are trying to do

- **Mindset:** stop thinking like a fad dieter. Think like a fit, healthy person. Fit, healthy people don't "suffer, eating healthy, boring foods". Instead, they "enjoy eating nourishing foods". They don't "force themselves to do boring exercise". Instead, they "enjoy training to hit their goals". You have to develop the mindset of a healthy person
- **Motivation:** you have got to want it enough to get through the tough bits. There will be hard times, hungry days, tough workouts, blood, sweat and tears (well, definitely sweat and tears) and you have to be motivated to keep pursuing the health and body you want enough to not give up
- **Emotional, psychological, social and spiritual support:** this is a tough one for a lot of people, because they may not have a supportive partner or family at home. In fact, sadly, this is far more common than you might think. People come to me with this problem a lot. An unsupportive or downright critical spouse can be a deal-breaker for a lot of people trying to reverse years of obesity and ill health. Some people have to handle a home or work environment where healthy living is ridiculed or rubbished, and that can really make life difficult. One of the reasons people join our 'club' *MND Life!* is for the community support, the networking with like-minded souls on a similar journey, the connection to a tribe

"Whether you think you can, or you think you can't, you're right."
- Henry Ford

The Mid-Levels

Once you have the foundations established in the Base Levels, you have the right **mindset**, you **want** change, you are **motivated,** you **believe in yourself** and you have a **supportive environment** established to keep you positive and encouraged, you are all set to start getting results. Now it's all coming together, this is where the action happens, this is the **major results zone.**

The middle third of the pyramid is largely about getting your body functioning efficiently, moving properly and fuelled correctly. This is all about gut function, physical structure, good habits, optimal nutrition and metabolism. It's about adjusting the MND lifestyle to be right for you, to eat right for your gut microbiome and your individual metabolism. Get these big pieces of the puzzle right, get everything working together, and this is where most of the results will come from.

- **Stop putting the wrong things in:** Core Principles 1 through 4 take care of this for you
- **Eat for nutrition, not for quantity:** many people in our culture are overfed but under-nourished. Don't be one of them. Core Principles 5 through 8 do this for you. It's all about nourishment
- Stop eating for **emotional support** and/or **entertainment.** If your spouse is an arsehole, talk to them, work through your problems together. Just hiding from the problem in comfort food won't fix anything, you'll just end up obese and self-loathing and *still* stuck in a shit marriage
- **Move more:** move naturally, create a habit of walking every day
- You might want to get a pet dog!
- Keep busy – **activity** is your friend. A full and busy life will help you not to 'boredom graze' your kitchen, or the local convenience store, and activity keeps your metabolism stoked and keeps you burning lots of calories
- **Reduce stress:** sort your life out, cut the things that are causing all your stress. Change your job if you are unhappy. Scale back, learn to live more modestly. Don't waste 20 years working a job you hate to pay for stuff that doesn't really make you happy
- Get better **quality sleep**, in a cool dark room, at night time. Get natural sunlight in the day, and sleep during the hours of darkness. If you work shifts, consider changing
- Establish a **daily exercise habit** – variety is the name of the game

The Top Levels

This really is the icing on the cake now, this is 'the details zone' where you tweak your individual version of the *Mother Nature's Diet* lifestyle to suit you.

This is all about optimisation of your ideal healthy lifestyle. Everything in this top section is making up 'the last 10% of the story.'

The Top Levels are just "the last 10% of the story" when it comes to weight loss and supreme good health, but interestingly, this is really **all the stuff that costs money.** This up here, in the last 5% to 10%, is **all the stuff they try to sell you**, all the stuff they advertise as "essential" or "life changing" or "amazing" or "must-have latest technology" and so on.

Buyer beware...

Optimisation of lifestyle

Think of all the stuff that so many companies are trying to sell you, such as these so-called superfoods, endless supplements promising the most amazing results, the latest stretchy Lycra clothing, fancy home-workout equipment, complex personalised diet and training programs, genetic tests, food intolerance testing, expensive detox retreats. That stuff is all relevant, I am sure it all plays a part, but you need to know that it is just detail, it's the last 10% at the top, **and it's all broadly pointless if you haven't sorted out the foundations below.**

- **Extra exercise:** once you are living a busy, active life, and you exercise most days, then adding more exercise on top will really only offer very minor additional benefits. Try to find sports and exercises you enjoy, and build in 40 to 60 minutes per day, ideally six days per week, even seven if you enjoy it, and keep your exercise varied, and consistent, and you'll be doing great
- **Spend more time outside**, during the day, especially when it is **sunny**. This all builds together; more activity, more walking, more exercise, more time outside and more time in the sunshine. That's not a list of five things, that's all one thing. Get outside for a walk every day and you are ticking all those boxes at once – and reducing stress while you are at it

- **Meal timing:** might be 5% of your success at most. The main advice would be to not eat your main meal of the day too late in the evening. Try to eat three hours before bed, give yourself time for digestion before you lie down
- **Genetics** might be 3% to 5% of the story. It may be 10% of the story (at most) if you are reading this book for cancer prevention, because you have all the risk factors and a family history. I remember attending a lecture with Professor Tim Spector, author and one of the UK's top genetics experts. I was chatting with him afterwards and asking him just how much genetics really matters in the bigger picture of the national obesity epidemic, the rise in diabetes, cancer prevention and more. His answer? 3%. Max. That's from the UK's top geneticist. Think of it this way: **your genes only load the gun; it's your lifestyle and diet that determine whether or not you pull the trigger**
- **Supplements and superfoods:** might be 1% to 2% of the story. Supplements play a more significant role in helping you to recover from specific deficiencies or conditions, but again if diet and gut function are not in order, their efficacy will be minimal. If you think you need supplements, consult with an expert first such as a Dietitian or Nutritional Therapist, don't just guess, as you'll likely end up wasting your money to make 'expensive urine'
- Expensive Lycra clothing, fancy gym kit, gadgets and apps – probably accounts for 1% to 2% of athletic ability, at best. A foundation of daily, varied exercise is key, don't get too lost in the gimmicks and 'latest thing' you see in the fitness magazines

Remember what this 'Pyramid of Success Factors' is trying to show you – it's the **relative importance** of these various factors, for your healthy living endeavours.

So, as an example, **consistency** is more important than what you eat or how you exercise. Why? Because you can have the most perfect healthy diet, the most perfect exercise schedule, the most perfect sleep patterns, time outside, sunshine, good hydration and low stress...but it's all completely pointless if it only lasts two weeks and then you go back to six months of binge drinking, late nights and junk food.

Consistency trumps everything else. You'll get better results on a mediocre diet and mediocre exercise plan if you maintain those habits 365 days of the year, than a perfect plan that only lasts a fortnight.

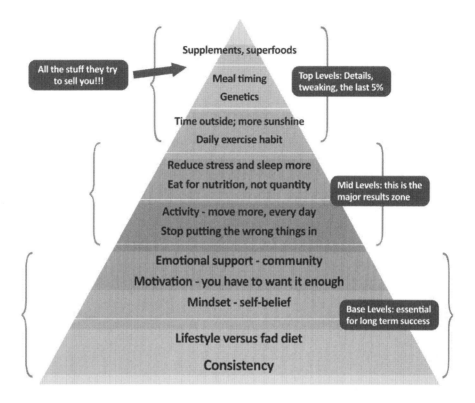

Flexibility

Is this all set in stone? No, of course not, the order of those labels may vary a little from person to person.

How come?

Because one size does not fit all.

Example, if you are a 55-yr old obese female with a family history of breast cancer, and you have habitually drunk too much for the last 30 years, then you may need to move "Genetics" way further down the pyramid, give it more focus, maybe take a DNA test, maybe hire me for a couple of coaching sessions and learn how best to set up your healthy lifestyle to start reducing and minimising certain risk factors. That's actually a great example of how the 12 Core Principles of *Mother Nature's Diet* work as a set of **broad guidelines**, *mostly* applicable to *most* people, but then *adjustable* for the *individual.*

Consistency versus snake oil salesmen

Consistency is king!!! Just remember that **the width of the pyramid indicates how important each factor is.** Consistency, lifestyle, mindset (not thinking like a fad dieter), self-belief, motivation and support are all *hugely important* to your success in weight loss and building your health and fitness. Buying the right 50 quid workout leggings, taking a ton of supplements and having a food intolerance test, these things are "minor details" by comparison.

Consistent lifestyle habits rule!! I would prefer you lay on the floor and do 10 sit-ups or crunches every day for a year, than do 500 one day and then nothing for a month. Men and their egos are terrible for this! I'm talking about the people who pack gyms in January only to leave them like a ghost town by March! That's fad diet mentality right there!

The genetic tests, supplements, superfoods and latest piece of home workout kit all have a place, and if recommended to you by a qualified professional who knows what they are talking about, they all doubtless have value – but the key here is to remember to *build your pyramid from the bottom up*! Get the **foundation factors in place first**, get into the results zone, get things moving and working and get momentum, then look at the latest protein supplements, genetic testing and superfoods as the final 10%, the last rungs of the ladder. Don't allow yourself to be distracted by expensive 'details' too early in the game – save your money for quality grass-fed meat and organic vegetables.

Important: Why is this here?

I want you to understand how the Pyramid of Success Factors fits in to the rest of this book. This whole book tells you what to do and why to do it. The 12 Core Principles and the 3 Key Lessons throughout this book, explain all you need to know.

The factors in The Pyramid, certainly in the Base Levels, are things you must sort out yourself, *you can't get them from this book*, **but you need them** to be successful.

The base levels

I don't mean to put a downer on anyone, but in all honesty, based on my own life experience and what I have seen in others over the last decade, without these things in place, long-term success is highly unlikely.

- **Consistency:** if you are 'on plan' for a week, then off for a month, that's yo-yo dieting. Some people do that for years. I did. For 20 years
- If you think this healthy eating malarkey is something you can do for 6 weeks to turn around 25 years of obesity, and then you can go back to the beer, the pizza and the ice cream, that's **fed diet behaviour**, and **it just doesn't work**
- If you don't **believe in yourself**, and you don't believe you can change, if you spend all your time telling yourself "I'm rubbish, I'm a failure, I will always be fat" then your chances of success are low
- **Motivation:** there will be hard times, there will be temptations, we live in an obesogenic world. There is a reason you got overweight in the first place – now you have to turn all that around. You have to be motivated, **you have to want to change.** If you *like* smoking and drinking and *you are comfortable* being obese and sedentary, then you are unlikely to make the effort required to change. That's not judgement, that's just the truth
- **You need support:** if your partner or spouse puts you down, insists on filling the house with sweets and chocolates, won't let you spend money on organics or gym fees, waves cakes and wine at you all the time...if your colleagues fill the workplace with cakes and biscuits...if your friends taunt you to quit 'this silly healthy eating thing' and constantly tempt you with booze and confectionery, then all these things make it much harder to create lasting changes in your eating and health habits. Our **MND Life! Membership Community** thrives, because we provide understanding, support, and a safe happy place for like-minded people

The frustrating reality is that you have to sort these things out first, in order to do everything else this book recommends that you do, to get the results you want. I think 99% of people I have ever met who struggle with yo-yo dieting, who struggle with sticking to healthy eating, or who have tried to live by the 12 Core Principles but not stuck it out, their 'failure' in that endeavour can be allocated to one of the factors listed on the previous page.

It's the difference between success and failure. It's that important.

The top levels

For so many people – that is people who don't have this book to guide them – when they start out on a weight loss drive or a healthy living regime, they direct a considerable proportion of their effort, attention, time and money at things that fall into the levels at the **top** of The Pyramid.

They make a New Year's Resolution to lose weight and get fitter, and the first thing they do is book up a week at a 'detox retreat' somewhere sunny. That's very nice – but get the basics in place first! It's great to go to a retreat for one week of the year, but not if your diet at home is crap the other 51 weeks, and you don't exercise regularly. You'll lose weight at the retreat then come straight home and put it on again!

I meet folks who loudly proclaim their grand new intentions to get in shape; to have 'visible abs by the summer'; or how they will look fantastic on the beach on holiday; they buy Lycra clothing, they buy every supplement known to man, they invest in swanky new £150-quid gel running shoes, and for about a week they share every health post going on Facebook, Instagram and Twitter, telling all the rest of us what latest wonderful superfood we should be having for breakfast. Then a fortnight later they give it all up!

By the time they are on that beach holiday in the summer, they've spent more time shopping for the gear and sharing posts on social media than they actually spent working out!

No, no, no! Epic fail! That's the world of fad diet mentality! They need to start with consistency...the foundation of The Pyramid...

Start at the bottom!
Work your way up!

For 90% of your journey, organic food and gym fees is all you need to spend money on, **at most**, and you can fund that by cutting out the booze (CP 4), the take away meals (CP 3) and the overpriced body sprays (CP 4).

- Be consistent
- Get support at home and at work, from friends and family
- Believe in yourself
- Know what you want, be motivated to hit your goals
- Clean up your diet (CP 1-4)
- Nourish yourself (CP 5-8)
- Move your butt, walk every day, get plenty of sleep (CP 9-12)
- Stick to it – the results will come

It's Not All Your Fault

In the opening pages of this book, back on Page 3 and 4, I noted that *Mother Nature's Diet* is all about taking personal responsibility, and working on yourself to get the best out of your life, in every way. Throughout the book I have constantly reiterated one of our core themes – **you have a choice.** You have more control over your health outcomes than you have been led to believe.

All of this drives home the point that it's down to you. If you are in great shape, you can pat yourself on the back, feel proud, and claim "I did that, that's all my own work." Equally, personal responsibility suggests that if you are in poor shape, you need to take it on the chin, face it, and go to work on yourself. It's your fault, you did it, not me, so quit complaining about it and get to work doing something about it.

*Well, actually, all of that is only **partly** true.*

You see, if you are in great shape and supreme good health, while you have doubtless worked hard to achieve that, you may also have had some help, and some luck, along the way.

- Perhaps you were gifted with **great genetics**; I doubt there is a successful model, accomplished ballet dancer, basketball star, Olympic athlete, champion jockey or competitive bodybuilder alive who would deny, that the hand they have been dealt from birth has been a crucial factor in determining their career choice
- Maybe you were lucky enough to come from loving, **supportive, proactive** parents, who taught you well, raised you to be fit and healthy and encouraged you in sport. Not all are so fortunate
- Or possibly you have been lucky enough to have **found you passion** for sport, or exercise, or weight lifting, or healthy eating, early in life, and did not fall foul of the trappings of a misspent youth, as many of us did in those early, impressionable years

And equally, on the other side of the coin, if you are in poor shape, while you may indeed have eaten the wrong things, eaten too much, drunk too much or failed to engage in regular exercise, that might not all be of your own *conscious choosing.*

- Maybe you have actually been trusting enough to follow the government **recommended dietary guidelines** that have been promoted in the UK from the end of the 1970s until now – to eat a diet based on a third or more of your food coming from starchy carbohydrates, including the white bread and white pasta shown on The Eatwell Plate, along with a further 12% or so of your diet from the sweets, cola drinks, cookies and chocolate also shown on The Eatwell Plate. Remember, for the first 15 years of the 21st century, they have been teaching The Eatwell Plate to school children in the UK, as part of the national curriculum
- Perhaps you have followed the crowd and believed the "eating fat gives you heart disease" story, along with the "eating fat makes you fat" story. I scarcely need to remind you that during the years this 'low fat, high-carb' dietary advice has been 'front and centre' here in the UK, obesity and type-2 diabetes **have both soared** to previously unprecedented epidemic levels
- Maybe you trusted the **food manufacturers**, the happy friendly brands made by Nestle, Coca-Cola, Kellogg's, General Mills, Mondelez and others, who offered us low-fat foods advertised as slimming options, while they were loaded with added sugars. Maybe you trusted those so-called "Heart healthy" low-fat spreads, the margarines containing potentially carcinogenic trans fats. Perhaps you trusted these companies as they invented **hyperpalatable foods**, *designed to make you eat far more than you needed*, placing food company profits before consumer health and wellbeing
- It could be that you followed those minimally-effective government guidelines on exercise, or you joined one of the UK's many well-known slimming clubs, that seem to promote severe calorie restriction yet offer little in the way of **food and nutrition education**. Diets that promote starving one day, to allow yourself 'treat points' for a cake the next, and diets that seem to base weight loss goals on some kind of perverse public **body-shaming**, weighing in front of each other once a week to either congratulate or berate each other on your success or failure

- Maybe you came from an upbringing that set you up for a lifetime of weight struggles from day one. That may be an unfortunate hand in the **genetics** pool; that may have been **poor food habits** inherited from your parents; or it may have been a **traumatic or unstable childhood** that created **emotional or disordered eating** into adult life

- Or possibly, despite the best will in the world, your home and work **environment** just make it incredibly hard to eat a diet high in fresh whole foods, and you are constantly bombarded daily with junk food, sugary snacks and confectionery. Today, many of our towns, universities, offices, motorway networks, rail networks and retail malls have become what is known as **obesogenic** environments

It is naïve and narrow-minded to just assume that everyone who is overweight and out of shape is just plain lazy. In many cases, they are. But in many cases, they are not.

For example, I can tell you right now, knowing my own body and metabolism as well as I do, and given my own history, I know beyond any shadow of a doubt, with my genetics (I have those so-called 'obesity genes' we read about in the press, I have had my DNA tested) that if I personally were to shift now to follow the precise dietary and exercise guidelines that our government recommend, I would shift in just a few months from my present 11% body fat into class 1 obesity, my fitness would decline, and my health would suffer.

I absolutely know beyond any doubt that if I were to live the next decade following a diet of 35%-40% starchy carbs and those minimal exercise guidelines the government recommend, that my weight would balloon and a year or two down the line I would shift back into obesity and likely stay there for the rest of my adult life.

I do preach **personal responsibility** here at *Mother Nature's Diet*, I do tell you it's down to you to take control of your own health and be responsible for your own health outcomes. But let's agree *not to play the blame game*. Let's draw a line under every day that has gone before today and say this is a fresh new start. **Because you can only take responsibility for your own outcomes, if you have been educated and given the right information in the first place.**

I think there are a lot of people out there who have unwittingly eaten themselves into a weight problem, or obesity, or type-2 diabetes, **without ever knowing they were doing anything wrong.**

I also think there are a lot of people out there who have eaten a lot of crap, drunk too many beers and been downright lazy. I can promise you that at almost every live seminar I have delivered over the last six years, people have come up to me in the break or at the end of the day and told me just that! *"I've been a lazy git and I admit it! Spending today with you has been the kick up the arse I needed to change my life!"*

So yes, there are a good few folks out there who have been gluttons and have been lazy, and they know it and admit it, but I think there are also **just as many** folks out there who have really tried to do the right thing, but our national dietary guidelines, and our misplaced trust in food manufacturers and supermarkets, have let these people down. **People need to know the truth, people need the correct knowledge in order to make the right decisions.**

People need the right education, to understand they have a choice.

- This book is that education
- You now have that knowledge
- Now you can take control
- Now **you have a choice**
- Your future is now under your control
- What's done is done. Forget the past. Let's start fresh from today
- Now...just start

There is a better way

You've looked at and learned about the 12 Core Principles. I want you to ask yourself this question:

What if he's right?

I took the grains, most of the starchy carbs and added sugars, almost all the processed foods, the alcohol and most of the chemicals out of my life; and I put the organic foods, 17-a-day vegetables and fruits, and a daily exercise habit in their place, and I lost 101 pounds of fat, 46 kilos or seven stone three.

I came off my medications, I went from fat to fit, I now have boundless amounts of energy, and libido, I've run a bunch of marathons, I don't take supplements, I don't take pills, I don't have an expensive gym membership, I don't have a home full of expensive gym equipment and I don't take any protein powders or other supplements.

I cured my own health conditions and came off my prescription medications, I'm doing my bit to help save our NHS because I'm in great shape, supreme good health. I haven't seen my doctor in years, I don't even know his or her name these days. I'm doing all I can to try to ensure I am ageing well and unlikely to 'become a customer in need' to the NHS any time soon.

Among those 847 books and studies I have read, and all those courses and seminars I have attended, I've studied the best diet to not get heart disease, the best diet to not have a stroke, the best anti-Alzheimer's diet, the best diet to avoid various types of cancer, the best diet to resist ageing, cognitive decline, dementia and Parkinson's. I have read books about the best diet to have more energy, the best diet for running marathons, the best diet for preventing type-2 diabetes, the best diet for managing type-1 diabetes, the best diet for weight loss, the best diet for bone health, mental health, to avoid depression, to avoid arthritis, gout, osteoporosis, you name it.

Add to all that books about agriculture, about mineral density in plants, animal welfare, avoiding soil erosion, I have visited farms, worked with farmers, learned about carbon sequestration, learned about dairy operations, attended lectures on greenhouse gas emissions. The list goes on and on. If there's a book about it, I've likely read it.

I've read about and learned about and studied all these different things, and **when you put them all together** and you ask "Well how can I do them all at once?" the answer is the **12 Core Principles** of *Mother Nature's Diet*.

I honestly and wholly believe, from my self-taught and self-experienced base of knowledge, that this is the best all-round preventive medicine, anti-ageing, high energy lifestyle I can give you after my three decades of learning. That's what you've got in this book.

Preventive medicine meets personal development.
Now you have the knowledge, it's down to you to apply it.

Lack of sex appeal

I am a pretty resilient chap, and I like a challenge, but I'll be the first to admit that after seven years now of promoting my message, selling common-sense healthy living advice to the British public is bloody hard work.

Preventive medicine just doesn't have the same sex appeal as "get a 6-pack". It's a hard sell.

Trying to get people to pay a few quid to attend my live seminars or join MND Life!, my monthly subscription-based healthy living 'club', for the purposes of learning common-sense based, no-bullshit, no-gimmick, preventive medicine is very hard work indeed. And yet, ask anyone who has just had a heart attack, or ask anyone who has just been diagnosed with cancer, if they could go back a decade or two and learn this stuff from the start, would they pay to learn the preventive medicine message?

Hell yeah, they'd pay anything to have that time over again, to have this knowledge, to do things differently and get back the healthy years they now face losing. **People only value their health, once it's gone.**

My mission in life is to get to them before the bad news comes their way. Christiaan Barnard, the pioneering heart transplant surgeon and author, famously said two things I wish to quote. He said...

"I don't believe medical discoveries are doing much to advance human life. As fast as we create ways to extend it, we are inventing ways to shorten it."

How true. According to the Christiaan Barnard Heart Foundation...In the last 10 years Prof. Barnard was intensively preoccupied with preventative medicine. His personal credo was:

"I saved the life of 150 people through heart transplantations. If I had cared about preventative medicine earlier, I would have saved 150 million people."

Indeed. I concur. **Prevention is better than cure.** *Mother Nature's Diet.*

The 28-Day Plan

E arlier in this book I wrote that with *Mother Nature's Diet* there is no highly-prescriptive 'Day One - eat x amount of this' or 'Day Two – do x amount of that' set regimen. **There can't be, because we are all different and one size does not fit all.** Over the following pages, I have provided a 28-Day Plan for you, it's as close to 'precise and prescriptive' as I can get, you'll have to adjust the details 'on the fly' according to your own circumstances.

That adjustment, how does that work? Well you are going to have to use some of that **common sense and personal responsibility** we have been talking about throughout the whole book! If the Plan says "scrambled eggs with spinach for breakfast" then you need to make scrambled eggs that are appropriate for you.

If you are a petite-built, 95-pound, 56-yr old female swimmer, you are going to want a smaller serving of scrambled eggs than if you are a heavy-built, 240-pound, 28-yr old male weight lifter. Adjust accordingly. One might have just two eggs, the other may want six eggs, and most of the rest of us are likely to land somewhere in between. Maybe three eggs is the right amount for you, or maybe for you it's four. If you are pretty active and you have come to MND looking for better health, more energy and muscle gains, then it's four. If you are less active and have come to MND looking for weight loss, then it's likely just two or three. You see? It's not so hard is it?

For this reason, where this 28-Day Plan gives recipes, you are not going to find details like "Add 150 grams of this to 30 grams of that, place in an oven at 160 degrees for 45 minutes" because all that is way too prescriptive. You are not going to read "Do 40 burpees, and 30 push-ups, then run three miles at nine-minute-miles pace" either. One person just read that last sentence and thought "Oh great, 40 burpees, 30 push-ups and a moderate-paced three-mile run, that sounds like great fun!" and another person read the same thing and though "Are you f*****g kidding me!! I haven't done 40 burpees in my lifetime never mind doing them in one workout!"

We are all different, so where the Plan says "do push-ups for one minute" then one person might manage 95 push-ups in perfect form, and another person might manage about seven or eight push-ups with their knees down.

Both is fine, if it means you are working at your pace, to your ability, and pushing yourself, then you are both doing it just right.

Over the following pages, I have detailed a 28-Day (four week) plan for you, and as I explain at the end, I actually suggest you do the whole thing twice – more on that later. Again, I have repeatedly explained throughout this book one size does not fit all and so it is pointless, misleading, and a complete waste of your time and mine, for me to lay out a single plan in great detail - I don't know you, the reader, and I cannot suggest precise detailed plan that will be perfect for you. You will have to adjust quantities and times and other details to make this work in your life, for your size, age, fitness, food preferences, and so on. Hopefully, reading this book, you have learned enough to make those small practical adjustments.

All that said, here are the key points to remember, how to live by the 12 Core Principles, in practical action points. You might like to think of this list as a kind of "*Mother Nature's Diet* Quickie Cheat Sheet" to help you get cracking as quickly as possible.

- Drop most of the processed grains and starchy carbs, and replace them with more vegetables instead
- Easy meal swaps -
    - Eggs for brekky, or fresh fruit, or bacon and egg, or a smoothie
    - Salad for lunch with smoked salmon, or flaked mackerel, tuna, hard boiled eggs, shredded ham, chicken or feta cheese
    - A chicken thigh, lamb chop or pork cutlet for dinner with lots of vegetables, or spaghetti Bolognese with broccoli instead of spaghetti
- Cut the cakes, biscuits, doughnuts, sweets, cookies, chocolate, fizzy drinks. If you feel you need a snack, have an apple. **Seriously, it's only 28 days of your life, come on now, you got this**
- Don't buy processed foods. Exercise restraint one time, in the supermarket, and you don't need to exercise restraint 50 times per week at home, because those foods won't be in your kitchen
- Better still, don't shop in a supermarket, seek out a local farm shop or farmer's market. Are there any local farms running an honesty box system for free-range eggs?
- Do you smoke? If so, you gotta quit. Can you do 28 days without? Can you talk to your GP about getting some help?

- Drink less booze – how about trying 28 days without a drink? If that scares you or seems like an unreasonably hard challenge, then I would encourage you to think about **your relationship with alcohol**. I was challenged to 30 days and that was where it all began for me. The thought terrified me! But I made 30 days (after the first week, it got much easier). Then later that year I did 90 days. The following year I tried 365 days…and here we are, over seven years now and I am still going, it's one of the best things I ever did for my own good health. And financially, I must have saved a small fortune by now!
- Makes sure you go outside every day for some fresh air. Ensure that a minimum of a 10-minute brisk walk becomes a non-negotiable part of every day. Just do it
- Drink at least eight to ten glasses of water every day, throughout the day
- Ensure 90% of your diet is comprised of fresh whole foods – plants and animals
- Buy organic, buy free-range, try to find grass-fed meat and dairy
- Exercise every day, even if it's just a walk
- Strength train a couple times per week
- Get a sweat going and your heart pounding a couple times per week
- Reduce stress – look at ways to pay off your debts, don't spend money you don't have, save and be sensible. Be loving, treat others as you would like to be treated
- Sleep more
- Get outside as often as you can – a few minutes every day, much more at the weekends
- Get it right 90% of the time. Then chill, everything will be OK

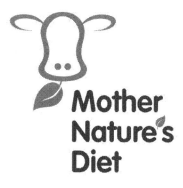

Week One

The Meals	Breakfast	Lunch	Dinner
Monday	Scrambled eggs with spinach, tomato on side	Salad with shredded ham or gammon	Chicken and roasted vegetables
Tuesday	Fresh fruit salad, including a few dark berries, spoonful of goat's yoghurt	Salad with feta cheese and red onion, drizzle with olive oil	Lamb steak with mixed steamed vegetables
Wednesday	Smoked salmon and a couple of eggs	Chicken salad with walnuts	Grilled fish with mixed steamed vegetables
Thursday	Breakfast smoothie	Salad with tuna fish	Stir fry (chicken, pork, beef, liver, kidney, or a mixture of three) and vegetables
Friday	No-grain pancakes with cinnamon	Ham and hard-boiled eggs on salad	MND chilli (no rice, veggies instead)
Saturday	Fish and greens. Sardines or mackerel with broccoli and kale	Homemade vegetable soup	Spaghetti Bolognese with broccoli or courgetti spaghetti
Sunday	Nut porridge with fresh berries	Sunday roast. Slow roasted shoulder of pork	Light meal or snack. Example, smoked salmon salad, or soup

The Exercise	Workout
Monday	Cardio 1
Tuesday	Strength training session 1
Wednesday	Bodyweight HiiT session 1. Or yoga class. Or favourite sport
Thursday	Cardio 2
Friday	Strength training session 2
Saturday	Bodyweight HiiT session 2. Or yoga class. Or favourite sport
Sunday	Nice long walk, try to add some hills

Note: the exercise descriptions are coming up after the meal plans.

Rules and goals for Week One (and the other weeks too!)

MEDICAL NOTE: If you are in poor health, taking medications, recovering from surgery, or you haven't exercised at all in many years, please do **check with your doctor** before you start a new exercise regime. If you take any medications, for anything, it's best to check with your doctor **before** you make substantial changes to your diet. Everything in this book is sound, there is nothing weird and whacky here, but it's best to check all the same, and I am sure your doctor will be delighted to know you are pushing into a pro-active, healthy lifestyle to improve your own health outcomes, rather than relying on medications.

Move naturally

As well as the exercise planned for each day, please make every possible effort to go out and walk every day, an additional walk. It might be just 10 minutes, maybe 20 minutes, or it might be an hour, it doesn't really matter how much, just please walk every day if you can.

Park a little further from the office, get off the bus or train a stop early, walk your dog in the morning before work, walk the kids to school, walk to the corner shop, just find an excuse to walk every day. Your Sunday workouts are planned as long walks, ideally a couple of hours or more. I am talking about in addition to the Sunday walk, the rest of the week please try to walk every day. If you develop a habit, like parking 15 minutes away from the office, you'll find you are adding that extra walk (there, and back, so that's 2 * 15 mins, daily) without any great effort. Unless it's tipping down with rain, then it will quickly become an effortless part of your regular routine, and you'll get quite used to it.

We *need* to do this, people in the UK walk 20% less now than we did a few decades ago, and it's contributing to all our obesity and health problems. Remember, if you want to lose weight, activity is your friend.

Sleep

You must get adequate sleep throughout the 28 days. If you are burnt out living on your nerves and surviving on five hours per night, you likely won't lose weight, won't feel better and will quit this plan feeling exhausted and blaming "that diet didn't work, just like all the others." Make sure you are getting seven or more hours every night. Eight or more will help with weight loss. Ensure your bedroom is cool, calm and properly dark. No night lights, no standby lights, no smartphones or tablets.

Water

As explained back in the chapters for Core Principle 5 and Core Principle 6, all too often people mistake the body's cries for fresh air and water as hunger pangs. Make sure you get fresh air every day – it goes with that daily walking habit we just talked about – and plenty of fresh water every day. Aim for eight to ten glasses per day, more if it's hot and you are sweating lots.

Feel free to skip a meal from time to time

Really, you won't starve. If you are skipping lunch, then I suggest a piece of fresh fruit and perhaps a small handful of almonds might keep you going. If you are skipping breakfast, not habitually but just from time to time, max once per week, then you don't need anything. This is, effectively, touching on another popular diet trend these days, **intermittent fasting (IF).** I'm not really covering that in this book, but if you want to try it, once a week, just skip breakfast, and go from finishing dinner the previous evening, by 7pm or 8pm, then not eating until 1pm the next day, then that's a nice little 17- or 18-hour fast, and you should feel fine and not be too troubled by hunger.

Is it healthy? Yes, it's quite a natural thing for your body to do.

How often? At this stage, max once per week is probably enough.

If you get a few hours into it and you are weak with hunger, and that hunger persists for some time, I suggest you are not ready for this yet, so have a piece of fruit, maybe a few nuts, and then eat well at your next meal. It's not for everyone. If you have been a 'sugar monster' or 'carbs addict', you'll find it harder, probably. When I do IF, I find a caffeinated coffee is all I need (or *like*, in truth, not *need*).

Meal plan notes

You'll notice that on weekends, where I have set Sunday lunch as a roast, I have then set dinner as a light snack. I'm just guessing you really don't need three big cooked meals in the space of 12 hours, that's just a lot of food!

In reality, you can be flexible at the weekends. For me personally, where I am usually up around 6am all week, I have an extra hour in bed at the weekend, and then I go walk my dog. It can easily roll around to 9am or 10am before I have my breakfast on Saturdays and Sundays, and then I just don't want or need another meal at lunchtime.

I find weekends are a good time to skip a meal, or just eat snack-sized meals. If we are eating a nice roast dinner as a family on Sunday, the rest of my day will be very small meals, or I'll use that as my day for extending my overnight fast through until lunchtime.

Experiment, do what feels right. The meal plans provided are guidelines, not a strict or detailed prescription. Enjoy!

28-Day Plan – FAQ's

Can I move things around?

Yes, absolutely, you can swap Monday for Thursday, Tuesday's workout on Saturday, Sunday's breakfast on Wednesday. Whatever it is, go for it. This plan is flexible in that way, so move stuff around to suit you, that is fine.

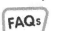
How do I prepare the meals?

There are a few recipes in the coming pages that explain roughly how to make the meals and what you need to know. These are not detailed, there is no fancy food or equally fancy professional photography. This Plan does not glorify food as if every meal you eat every day of your life should look like something from a photo-shoot. The real world isn't like that. If you want that you'll need to buy some fancy recipe books.

This plan puts food in context with the rest of your life. The meals are straight forward, not so mouth-wateringly delicious that you will want to overeat, but tasty enough to keep you happy and satisfied. The focus is on nutrition, not on quantity or taste sensations. This whole Plan is pretty much how I live all the time, real world stuff, it's designed to work for a busy professional or busy family person, it's all fairly quick and simple.

Can I have a cheat day?

Well, you're only cheating yourself. The whole plan is only 28 days of your life. If you have likely been eating the wrong things and not moving enough for ten years, that's already 3652 cheat days in the bag, can't you manage 28 without another one?

Can I drink tea and coffee?

Yes, you can, but no milk and sugar. For more on coffee and caffeine, see my blog FAQs[1]. I suggest finding herbal teas that you like – lemon and ginger, mint, raspberry, camomile, there are a gazillion teas out there, find a couple you like and stock up.

Why have you not given me 28 different breakfast recipes and 28 different lunch recipes for 28 different days?

Holy moly, did you actually read the rest of the book? Are we even on the same wavelength?

---

[1] *Mother Nature's Diet* blog, FAQs:
https://mothernaturesdiet.me/2016/09/16/mother-natures-diet-faqs-is-it-healthy-to-drink-coffee/

When I meet folks who eat sugar-coated cereal for breakfast and white-bread sandwiches for lunch, they seem happy to eat virtually the exact same thing day-in, day-out, week-in, week-out for years and years on end and they never complain they are bored and they never ask for variety. Suggest they eat healthily, and suddenly they are terribly bored and complaining that this healthy eating lark is dull. Funny, that.

Maybe it's because the cereal and sandwiches are artificially sweetened to make you love them and crave them, that's part of the reason why you got overweight in the first place, remember? The real food is natural, and you won't crave it the same way – good, this might help you to stop over eating. Additionally, the years of processed food very likely 'damaged' your palate; your taste buds came to believe everything should taste sweet until dinner, then you like to put hot chili sauce on your food. Now you need to 'retrain' your taste buds to get off their 'sugar poisoning', and get back to tasting real fresh whole foods. Let's try 28 days as a starter and see if that helps!

Do I have to follow the workout plan precisely?

No, you don't. The training plans here fit with the ethos of MND Core Principle 9. You have cardio twice weekly, strength training twice weekly, bodyweight HiiT-style training twice weekly and a 'rest day' for getting out on a long walk. Feel free to move it all around throughout the week to suit you.

What is HiiT training?

Home based, no-equipment-required, easy HiiT training is the simplest thing to do. HiiT means High Intensity Interval Training – it's a type of training that is proven to give you a good workout in a short space of time, burning lots of calories and getting your heart rate racing and engaging lots of your muscles all at once. It's 'all the rage' these days, and that's a popularity that is well deserved, because HiiT training is a highly effective tool that anyone can use to maintain and increase strength, burn fat and boost fitness all at once.

HiiT routines are typically short, they typically involve short bursts of activity and short rests repeated over the duration of the workout. Anyone can do HiiT at home, without any special equipment, any time, any place – at home, in the house, in the garden, in the park, on the beach, anywhere. It's fast, furious and fun!

Week Two

The Meals	Breakfast	Lunch	Dinner
Monday	No-grain pancakes or banana and egg scramble	Leftover pork with vegetables, stir fry	Chicken with a fresh green salad
Tuesday	Sausage and egg, with greens, fresh tomato on the side	Salad with leftover roast pork	Homemade vegetable soup and goat's cheese on the side
Wednesday	Omelette (add mushrooms, ham, salmon, what you fancy)	Tuna and red onion salad with a little feta cheese	Roasted Mediterranean vegetables (vegetarian tonight)
Thursday	Breakfast smoothie (or juice) or soup for a cold day	Mackerel or tuna salad	Lamb steak with roasted vegetables
Friday	Scrambled eggs and green veggies (spinach, kale, broccoli)	Chicken or gammon on a salad	Grilled fish with steamed vegetables
Saturday	Fresh fruit salad with a few nuts, spoonful of goat's yoghurt	Bowl of soup or a light salad, your choice	Spaghetti Bolognese – MND-style broccoli Bolognese
Sunday	Full English – bacon, sausage, eggs, tomato, mushrooms	Sunday roast, chicken and vegetables	Homemade vegetable soup and goat's cheese on the side

The Exercise	Workout
Monday	Cardio 1
Tuesday	Strength training session 1
Wednesday	Bodyweight HiiT session 1. Or yoga class. Or favourite sport
Thursday	Cardio 2
Friday	Strength training session 2
Saturday	Bodyweight HiiT session 2. Or yoga class. Or favourite sport
Sunday	Nice long walk, try to add some hills

Week Three

The Meals	Breakfast	Lunch	Dinner
Monday	Scrambled eggs with spinach, tomato on side	Leftover chicken with salad	Gammon and roasted vegetables
Tuesday	Fresh fruit salad, including a few dark berries, spoonful of goat's yoghurt	Salad with feta cheese and red onion, drizzle with olive oil	Lamb steak with mixed steamed vegetables
Wednesday	Smoked salmon and a couple of eggs	Chicken salad with walnuts	Grilled fish with mixed steamed vegetables
Thursday	Breakfast smoothie	Tuna and red onion salad with Feta cheese	Slow-cooker chicken and vegetables
Friday	Nut porridge with fresh berries	Gammon and hard-boiled eggs on salad	Chilli-con-carne (MND-style, no rice, veggies instead. Add some liver too! See *)
Saturday	Fish and greens. Sardines or mackerel with broccoli and kale	Homemade vegetable soup	MND ham, egg and 'chips'
Sunday	No-grain pancakes with cinnamon	Sunday roast – shoulder of lamb	Light meal or snack. Example, smoked salmon salad, or soup

* Note from previous page: You could try adding some liver, diced up finely, with the minced beef, in your chilli, just chop it up small and mix it in and then cook the chilli dish. Basically, add some liver and hope the kids don't notice! Sneak those extra nutrients in!

The Exercise	Workout
Monday	Cardio 1
Tuesday	Strength training session 1
Wednesday	Bodyweight HiiT session 1. Or yoga class. Or favourite sport
Thursday	Cardio 2
Friday	Strength training session 2
Saturday	Bodyweight HiiT session 2. Or yoga class. Or favourite sport
Sunday	Nice long walk, try to add some hills

Week Four

The Meals	Breakfast	Lunch	Dinner
Monday	No-grain pancakes or banana and egg scramble	Leftover lamb with vegetables, stir fry	Chicken and roasted vegetables
Tuesday	Fresh fruit salad with a few nuts, spoonful of goat's yoghurt	Salad with feta cheese, red onions, apple, celery and sultanas	Slow-cooker pork chops with mixed vegetables
Wednesday	Fish and greens, sardines or mackerel, broccoli and kale	Mackerel or tuna salad	Grilled fish with a large salad or roasted vegetables
Thursday	Omelette (add mushrooms, ham, salmon, what you fancy)	Chicken or gammon on a salad	Lamb cutlet with roasted vegetables
Friday	Scrambled eggs, with spinach and feta cheese, possibly smoked salmon on the side	Your choice of salad, any topping, or soup on a cold day	Chicken and roasted vegetables
Saturday	Sardines or pilchards with eggs and greens	Bowl of soup or a light salad, your choice	Curry (MND-style, no rice, veggies instead)
Sunday	Banana and egg scramble with sultanas and cinnamon	Sunday roast – beef or wild game from local butcher	Homemade vegetable soup and goat's cheese on the side

The Exercise	Workout
Monday	Cardio 1
Tuesday	Strength training session 1
Wednesday	Bodyweight HiiT session 1. Or yoga class. Or favourite sport
Thursday	Cardio 2
Friday	Strength training session 2
Saturday	Bodyweight HiiT session 2. Or yoga class. Or favourite sport
Sunday	Nice long walk, try to add some hills

The recipes

Honestly, I think it's a flaw of so many 'weight loss books' when they give you pages and pages of wonderful sounding recipes with fabulous professional photographs that make all the meals look and sound absolutely delicious. *I'm trying to get my readers to eat a little less*, not salivate over all the fab looking dishes that they can't wait to try out!

Also, I think that a bunch of complex recipes just adds extra effort to the whole thing. "Oh, the recipe said 35 grams of such-and-such, I can't get that in my local shops, can I use blah-blah instead?" and "It says chicken today but I don't really like chicken, I have really been enjoying the fish dishes, I wish I could have fish again this evening."

Yes!! OK, have the fish!

Seriously, no drama, the meal plans I have set out for you over the previous pages are a handy guide, not a set of commandments issued by Royal Decree on pain of death! The thing is, over the last five or six years, I find there are two types of people. Some want exact details, they want to be told what to eat, when to eat it, how to prepare it, every detail laid out. Others, get stressed out if the details are too prescriptive, and wish the diet plan offered more flexibility to adapt to their work and life routine. No book, this book included, will ever please everyone in both groups.

Therefore, what you have in these pages is a guide, not a prescription. I am suggesting enough detail to meet the needs of the first group, but leaving the details open enough to allow the latter group the flexibility they yearn for. Well, that's my intention, I hope you find it works.

Meal basics: A main meal should contain a palm-sized portion of protein, and then heap the plate with veggies or salad. That's so easy!

How to cook: I'm not going to tell you how to cook scrambled eggs in great detail with weights and times and temperatures. Three minutes at 200 degrees this, add so many grams of that for two minutes. I mean, come on, really, just stick a knob of butter in a pan, heat it up, crack in a few eggs, throw in a couple of handfuls of spinach, stir it around for a few minutes and serve. Really, do we need to go into four pictures and a step-by-step plan for that? Same for a stir fry. Chop everything up, chuck it in a frying pan or wok, stir fry it around for ten minutes. Seriously, it's that easy.

I'm not being facetious, that's just how I cook. Honestly, I don't think I have ever followed a detailed recipe in my life. The only specific recipe I have ever written in my life is for my own *MND Moroccan lamb*, and oh boy it is so good! Do try it (Week Three, Sunday!) Yummy![2] All that said, following are some basic guidance notes to help you get cracking.

A few specifics

No-grain pancakes (alternative: banana and egg scramble)

Pancakes for breakfast are an old favourite for many people, but obviously we don't make our pancakes with flour the way most people do. MND grain-

---

[2] *Mother Nature's Diet* blog, see: https://mothernaturesdiet.me/2013/07/06/moroccan-spiced-slow-roast-lamb/

free pancakes use bananas and eggs, and they are super-simple, super-quick and super-tasty. I can't remember where I first heard of this recipe, but I've I have been making this for years, it's a staple of the Paleo crowd, and it's surprisingly very popular these days.

Start with one large banana to two eggs, and increase the quantity in that ratio if you want more. These quantities are pretty flexible – sometimes I add more bananas, sometimes more eggs, it all seems to work out OK. Mash the banana(s) into a bowl on its own first, and then mash the eggs into the banana. Heat a knob of butter in a pan, dollop the mix in, and quickly fry the mix like a pancake for a few mins, both sides, job done.

I like to add a handful of sultanas, but that's optional – my kids won't eat the sultanas, they seem to think they are rabbit poops, so I leave them out for the kid's breakfast. You can spread the whole mix out and make 1 big pancake, or drop it into the pan in dollops and make several small pancakes, and you can add more eggs to thin it out, or more banana to thicken it up.

Sometimes, rather than making several small pancakes, I just mix it all together in the bowl and then drop the lot into the warm pan in one go and stir-fry it around to make 'banana scrambled eggs' or 'banana and egg scramble' which works better if your non-stick pan, well, sticks. You may like to add those sultanas and sprinkle a good dash of cinnamon on top too, it's absolutely delicious.

Stir-fry leftovers for lunch

Really, this is the quickest and easiest thing, I eat this way at least twice a week for lunch. It barely needs writing up.

I always cook more at the weekends than we need as a family. If I need to buy a two-kilo shoulder of pork to feed us all a Sunday roast, I'll buy the three-kilo shoulder instead, and then I have enough leftovers for several additional meals.

Lunchtime leftovers – grab my pan, start with a smear of butter or lard, grab a bunch of seasonal veggies, rough chop them up, thrown them in on the heat. Grab a serving of leftover meat or fish or whatever I have, throw that in too. Add a little seasoning, some herbs and/or spices, stir fry it around for a few minutes, and we are done.

Lunch in 10 minutes. Never the same meal twice. Literally, never the same. Chili and lime. Coriander and lime. Paprika, cumin, ginger and cinnamon. Cinnamon, apple and sultanas. Rosemary and garlic. There are endless choices for flavourings. I grow both veggies and fresh herbs in my garden, so I use whatever is seasonal and fresh.

Homemade vegetable soup

This is delicious and simple. On days when lunch was large and you only need a light evening meal, a bowl of homemade vegetable soup is spot on. Or use as a warming breakfast or lunch on a cold winter's day.

Start with a big saucepan (make sure it's one with a lid) and drizzle in a little olive oil. Chop up an onion (I use red onions, personal preference) and throw that in first. Chop up half of a butternut squash (you have to peel it first) into cubes and throw that in. Season with black pepper. Whack the heat up full, it'll start sizzling after a minute, then stick the lid on and turn it down to simmer heat for about 15 mins.

While it simmers, boil the kettle and make 1.5 litres of stock – we use low-salt Bouillon, it's one of the healthiest stock options out there, with few artificial additives in it. If you want to go "hard core" on me you can use just water but it makes the soup a bit tasteless, so then you'll need to use some extra herbs for seasoning. After these 15 mins, add the Bouillon and about 100 grams or more of fresh spinach, turn up the heat a bit and cook for five or ten minutes.

That's it, finished. I suggest leaving it to cool for a while (then re-heat afterwards) before you blend it, as hot liquids, poured into a jug style blender, tend to expand – I've done the whole "re-decorate the kitchen with green splattered exploding hot soup" trick and it's not so great to be honest. However, if you don't want to wait, then use a handheld blender and just blend the soup in the pan.

For some variety – just experiment. You can vary these soups like crazy. Swap out the spinach for courgettes, which are great in soup, or use 2 carrots with half a squash. You can use kale, or rocket or watercress instead of spinach, or all of them, bell peppers are not so good, and you can use parsnips, beets, turnips.

The butternut squash is the main thing, or you can switch that for a large sweet potato. Carrots and pumpkin also make perfect bases for homemade soup. You can adjust the quantity of the stock to suit the thickness you like. I like thick soups, so we never put too much stock in.

Roasted vegetables

Many of the evening meals in the 28-Day Plan are based around a small serving of protein (a chicken thigh or breast, a lamb cutlet or steak, a pork chop, a couple of slices of gammon, or grilled fish) served with a good heap of mixed, seasonal, roasted vegetables.

In a large casserole or oven-proof dish, dice up your choice of veggies. Sweet potato, butternut squash, raw beetroot, carrots and parsnips – these starchy root veggies need an hour in a medium heat oven. The softer vegetables – onions, cherry tomatoes, courgettes, bell peppers, mushrooms, cauliflower, leeks, broccoli (beware, it burns easily) all only need half an hour.

Set the oven to a medium heat, around 175 degrees, stir your veggies around with some extra virgin olive oil and herbs for seasoning, a sprinkle of Himalayan rock salt and some black pepper, and in they go.

I usually do the squash or sweet potato first, with any other root veggies, then after half an hour, throw in the rest and give it all a stir around in the warm oil to keep it all moist. At that half hour stage, I put the meat or chicken in too, in the same oven, in a separate dish. Around half an hour is about right to oven bake the meat. Voila, the whole meal is ready, quick and easy. Tops 15 minutes prep time, then an hour cooking, and it's all ready.

This meal ticks all the MND boxes – a palm-sized serving of protein filling a quarter to a third of your plate, then the rest of your meal is veggies. It packs up to six of seven servings of veggies depending on the size of your meal. It loads in veggies of different colours so you get different nutrients, and it's delicious! Winner!

You can add a smear of pesto sauce, tomato puree, chili sauce, herbs, spices to the meat or fish, if you need to, add whatever you like to add flavour. If I have chicken breast, sometimes I add a smear of pesto sauce (just a tiny bit) or tomato puree and a dash of herbs just to add flavour. Most any other meat or fish option I don't bother. I just find chicken breast rather dry and bland on its own (another good reason why I prefer thigh meat.)

Salads

You can do almost anything you like with salads. Some people like a really plain salad, just some lettuce shredded, a tomato or two, not too much else. Some people love to add a million ingredients and make their salad a vibrant explosion of colour. What you do, is up to you. You may use a variety of greens (lettuces, spinach, rocket, watercress), various types of tomatoes, bell peppers, raw mushrooms, cooked beetroot, cucumber, pickles, nuts and seeds (careful on the extra calories), celery, grated carrot, coleslaw, olives, sultanas, avocado, olive oil or salad dressing. Go steady on the added oils, nuts and seeds and avocado, these things will ramp up the extra calories fast, so beware of that if weight loss is your primary goal.

The list goes on and on, you can make up your salads how they suit you, and your guide should be: make it varied and tasty enough to keep you interested, and to enjoy eating a variety of textures and colours, which should ensure you get a variety of nutrients, but don't make it so colourful, so artistic and delicious, that you are tempted to overeat!

MND ham, egg and 'chips'

The MND version of 'ham, egg and chips' is delicious. Roasted gammon or ham, sliced up, boiled new potatoes with butter and herbs, hard-boiled eggs (shelled of course), and a big salad. Ham, egg and 'chips' the healthy way!!

Breakfast smoothie

Your 28-Day Plan includes a smoothie as a breakfast option once each week (for 3 weeks). If you don't own a blender or you just don't want a cold liquid breakfast, that's fine, repeat one of the other breakfasts instead.

If you do own a blender, or Nutri-Bullet or Ninja or whatever those things are called, then you can make a smoothie easily. Just add a couple of pieces of fruit, a couple of vegetables, and something like some almond milk, blend it all up, and you are good to go. Experiment with what works for you, or visit my blog site at www.mothernaturesdiet.me and try some of the smoothies mentioned in various posts on there. My old stock favourite – 1 large carrot, 1 large banana, a small handful of cashews, a raw egg or two, blended up with almond milk, and a handful of spinach.

Nut porridge

First off, I have to admit that this breakfast option is not for those on a tight budget. It can also pack a lot of calories, so don't underestimate this meal!

From time to time I buy lots of bags of nuts from my local whole foods store – almonds, hazelnuts, Brazils, walnuts, pecans and sometimes cashews. Buy all the natural ones, none of those salted or sweetened nuts obviously. I crush/grind the lot in my little blender/grinder and then mix them all together in a sealed storage container (like a Tupperware box or similar).

This is then ready to go in the kitchen cupboard any time I want it. Making nut porridge for breakfast is then as quick and easy as can be. **Just a few spoonsful** of this lovely (and **highly calorie dense**!) nut mix in a cereal bowl, and add a little liquid of your choice, and you are ready to go. You can add cold water, warm water, nut milk, goat's milk, or grass-fed dairy milk. Alternatively, you may want to moisten this with a spoonful or organic yoghurt (I use goat's milk yoghurt) or a dash of heavy cream. Top with sliced apple and fresh berries, or any other fruit of your choice.

Other meals listed

Where the plan shows 'lamb steak with steamed vegetables' I don't think you need a recipe for that. Just grill or oven bake a lamb steak or cutlet, and pick a selection of vegetables to steam. Don't fancy lamb? Have a pork chop or chicken thigh. Don't have a steamer? Boil those veggies instead. It's all quite quick and easy – the meat needs 15 to 20 minutes under the grill, or half an hour in the oven, and the veggies need 15 minutes in the steamer, and you're all done.

Sunday roasts

I'm leaving you to do a roast as you normally would. Personally, I like my shoulder of pork super slow roasted for six hours (I use a Jamie Oliver recipe you can find online or in his books) and I like to do lamb either in rosemary and garlic, or MND Moroccan style as mentioned previously. You do your roast how it suits you – skip the Yorkshire puddings and go easy on roast potatoes – just have a couple!

For the other meals listed in the plan, you already know what to do:

Spaghetti Bolognese. Just make the Bolognese sauce as you normally would (add some veggies to the mix if you like) and then serve with broccoli, courgetti spaghetti or cauliflower instead of spaghetti.

Chili-con-carne or curry. Just make the meat and sauce as you usually would, ideally making your own from scratch blending the spices, rather than using a store-bought sauce. Then serve with vegetables instead of rice. Chili goes well with broccoli or cabbage, and curry goes great with cauliflower, in my opinion, but experiment to find what works for you. Cooking a chili or a curry is a great opportunity to add some liver or kidneys to a meal and hope the family don't notice! If your kids are like mine, and don't want to eat liver, chop some up fine and add it to a chili or curry and they'll never notice.

Snack options

You don't need a ton of snacks...the goal is to cut back and lose weight, remember. If you are eating proper-sized, healthy, nutritious meals, then you really should be quite comfortable going four or five or six hours between meals without eating. Check that any hunger pants are not in fact cries for air or water or some movement and exercise. But if you are genuinely hungry and you must eat between meals, try these options:

- Fresh fruit – apple, pear, orange, satsuma, grapefruit, clementine, a few berries
- Nuts and seeds – a few almonds, plain cashews, walnuts. Pumpkin seeds. But go easy, the calories soon add up
- Carrot sticks, cucumber sticks, celery, sliced up bell peppers, spring onions, dipped in hummus, but go steady, the calories can add up
- Water, and air, remember – don't fall victim to false hunger pangs. Be sure you are not just bored!

Shopping list basics

This is not an exhaustive list. Your list will vary according to how many people in your household, what's available where you live, the climate and season, and your individual likes and needs. This list is just a few basics to remember, these items should ideally form the majority of your weekly food shop.

Vegetables

- Broccoli and kale
- Carrots
- Parsnips
- Spinach, chard
- Peppers

- Cucumber
- Mushrooms
- Cabbage, cavolo nero, spring greens
- Cauliflower
- Courgettes
- Onions
- Sweet potatoes, pumpkin, squash
- Salad leaves
- Tomatoes
- Avocado (I know, it's a fruit!)

Meats

- Pork
- Chicken
- Lamb
- Organ meats – liver, kidneys
- Wild game, based on seasonal and local availability
- Beef or beef mince

Seafood

- Smoked salmon
- Fresh sardines
- Mackerel
- Tinned tuna (pole and line caught, MSC stamped) (or fresh tuna steaks if you can get them)
- Pilchards
- Trout or other freshwater fish as available
- Catch of the day - cod? What does your fishmonger have?
- Shellfish (no allergy?)

Fruits

- Apples
- Bananas

- Pears
- Oranges
- Satsumas or clementines
- Grapefruit
- Seasonal berries
- Lemons
- Plums

Other

- Free-range eggs
- Grass-fed butter (can you find a butter made from unpasteurised milk?)
- Extra-virgin olive oil (perfect world = cold, pressed once)
- Organic dark chocolate (75% to 90%)
- Fairtrade organic coffee (organic is important, so is Fairtrade. Growing coffee beans uses a ton of pesticides, and over the years, many coffee farmers in the tropics have been among the most unfairly treated farmers of any crops, so please, shop Fairtrade for the farmers, and shop organic for your health)
- Nuts – almonds, walnuts, plain cashews
- Feta cheese (made from goat's milk)
- Goat's yoghurt
- Herbal tea bags (lemon and ginger, mint tea, camomile, green teas, fruit teas, there are so many to chose from)
- Olives
- Pumpkin seeds (scoop from fresh pumpkin and roast yourself?)
- Herbs and spices
- Dried fruits (dates, sultanas)
- Organic artisan cheese (try some Parmigiano Reggiano or French Comté cheese for a natural, grass-fed, healthy option)
- Almond milk or coconut milk
- Hummus

The exercises

I want you to really enjoy your training sessions, so I have provided you with a nice variety of exercises, and it all fits in with our goals outlined in Core Principle 9.

- Twice per week cardio
- Twice per week weights/strength training
- Twice per week bodyweight HiiT style training – you can swap this to a sport you enjoy. Rugby? 5-a-side footy? Hockey? Horse riding? Yoga? This is meant to be fun!
- Sundays are for long walks. Get your spouse or family out with you, make it fun time together out in nature

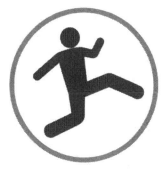

MEDICAL NOTE - REPEATED: If you are in poor health, taking medications, recovering from surgery, or you haven't exercised at all in many years, **please do check with your doctor before you start a new exercise regime.** If you take any medications, for anything, it's best to check with your doctor before you make substantial changes to your diet. Everything in this book is sound, there is nothing weird and whacky here, but it's best to check all the same, and I am sure your doctor will be delighted to know you are pushing into a pro-active, healthy lifestyle to improve your own health outcomes, rather than relying on medications.

What's the goal?

If you are a **complete beginner**, the cardio sessions are intended to elevate your heart rate, get you using your lungs, get your diaphragm moving, make you puff and pant a bit and break a sweat. If you are **already used to training**, then these sessions should be pushing you to *improve your fitness*.

For **absolute beginners**, the strength training sessions are designed to stimulate your muscles to start doing some work. At first, we are looking to stop age-related loss of strength and loss of range of motion, then in time, you will be looking to start increasing strength and muscle mass. For more **intermediate and the advanced**, these sessions should be more challenging, pushing you to *make gains in strength and muscular endurance.*

The bodyweight HiiT-style workouts are fun! They make you move, you get some fitness benefits, and some strength and muscular endurance gains. They are designed to make you puff, pant, sweat, bend and stretch!! Enjoy!!

You'll see **cardio twice weekly** – over the 28 days, you can mix those sessions up if you want to, some swimming, jogging, cycling, or gym-based cardio such as indoor rower, treadmill, stepper or elliptical trainer, whatever you enjoy. So maybe 'Cardio 1' might be swimming, and 'Cardio 2' might be cycling. **It's your week, you make it work for you.** If you enjoy one type of cardio only, such as running, cycling or swimming and you want to do that for all your cardio sessions, that's fine then, do that. It's all about you being happy and enjoying yourself.

It's the same story with the **strength training** and **HiiT sessions**. If you have come to *Mother Nature's Diet* overweight and out-of-shape and it's all new to you, pitch in at beginner's level and start gently, doing the best you can and looking to improve over the 28 days as we go.

But if you are a seasoned athlete and you have come to MND looking to improve your diet, tighten up that midsection, or address your health concerns, then you likely already know what you are doing here, and you can continue your own training regimen if you like. (That is, of course, providing your training regimen is balanced, varied, healthy, and it's working for you! If it's not any of those things, then perhaps you should try following mine?)

If you have a **favourite sport** you like to play, or enjoy working on strenuous jobs in the garden, you can substitute some of the HiiT sessions accordingly. If you decide to join a yoga class, that can substitute for the bodyweight training session too.

Just make sure you are moving your body, pushing yourself at whatever level means 'push' to you, and having fun at the same time.

With all the strength training sessions and HiiT-style workouts, don't expect miracles from day one. If you are a beginner, **just start**, do the best you can, and look to improve a little each time from session to session. If you can't squat all the way down so that your thighs go down to parallel with the floor, then just do what you can and try to make improvements each week. If you can't do full push-ups, that's OK, put your knees down and build up the strength.

Buy some little dumbbells or hand-weights (lots of places online to order from, such as Amazon or many others, they should only cost ten or twenty pounds, you don't need to spend a fortune) to hold for the strength training sessions – for bicep curls, shoulder presses and triceps kickbacks. If you don't know what these exercises are, just type "How to do ___" into YouTube and you'll find demonstrations for each one – there is not space for dozens and dozens of pictures of all the exercises in this book.

Rope in a friend or family member to train with, give each other encouragement and moral support, egg each other on and hold each other accountable to get through the 28 days together as a team. That's our MND week – a couple of cardio sessions, a couple of strength sessions, a couple of mixed bodyweight sessions, a long walk at the weekend and a short walk as often as possible. This 28-Day Plan puts it all together for you.

Beginner's workouts

Cardio workout plan for beginners: those totally unaccustomed to doing any exercise at all. These are your 'cardio sessions' as noted on the schedule.

Week	Activity	Duration	Intensity
1	Walking	2 sessions @ 30 mins	Moderate pace
2	Brisk walking	2 sessions @ 40 mins	Brisk pace, try to find some hills if you can
3	Interspersed light jogging and walking	2 sessions @ 50 mins	Just what you feel capable of, moderate effort
4	Interspersed light jogging and walking	2 sessions @ 60 mins	Push a little harder, moderate to hard effort

Strength training workout for absolute beginners. Where the schedule on Page 235 (and the following pages for Week Two, Three and Four) shows "Strength training session 1" or "Session 2" these are the workouts to use.

Movement	Weight	Repetitions	Notes
Prisoner squats	Bodyweight, can hold extra weights as you progress	12 to 20	Go slow and low
Push-ups	Bodyweight	10 to 20	Use knees if required
Standing knee raises with hold	Bodyweight	20	Each leg
Lunges	Bodyweight	20	Each leg
Shoulder overhead press	Use weights to your ability	10	Both sides
Shoulder side raise	Use weights to your ability	10	Both sides
Shoulder front raise	Use weights to your ability	10	Both sides
Biceps curls	Use weights to your ability	20	20 each arm
Triceps kickbacks	Use weights to your ability	10 to 20	Reps each arm
Chair dips	Bodyweight	10 to 15	Ensure chair stable
Calf raise on step	Bodyweight	10 to 15	Hold wall for stability
Standing touch toes	Bodyweight	1 minute	Stretch

Bodyweight HiiT Plan for complete beginners. Where the schedule on Page 235 (and the others...) shows "Bodyweight HiiT session 1" or "Session 2" these are the workouts to use.

Movement	Work time	Rest time	Notes
Prisoner squats	30 seconds	30 seconds	Back straight
Push-ups	30 seconds	30 seconds	Use knees if required
Crunches or sit-ups	30 seconds	30 seconds	Not sit ups if you suffer low back pain
Burpees	30 seconds	30 seconds	Lunges (alternative)
Squat thrusts	30 seconds	30 seconds	Old school!
Jump squats*	30 seconds	30 seconds	They are hard!

* That's a squat down, and explosive jump up, feet leaving the ground on every jump. Oh, go on, it's only 30 seconds! Just mind your knees!

There you go, just 6 minutes. Take a minute to rest, then see if you can do it again. Beginners, your targets to shoot for:

- During week 1, can you complete 2 rounds of this in 15 minutes?
- During week 2, can you complete 3 rounds, in 20 minutes?
- During week 3, can you get through 4 rounds, in 30 minutes?
- During week 4, can you make it 5 rounds in 30 minutes?

Exercise notes

Strength training routine: Aim to complete the whole thing in about 15 minutes. Focus on form, not speed. If this is all completely new to you, then I would suggest you could start with just 15 minutes each day, and progress up to 20, then 30 minutes (the whole circuit twice).

Bodyweight HiiT: Do the best you can! Enjoy it, have a laugh, it's meant to be fun. If you can't do push-ups, put your knees down and build up the strength. It will come in time. Beware of putting your hands too wide apart for push-ups, that can cause shoulder injuries for some people.

Intermediate workouts

Cardio workout plan for those with **intermediate** ability and experience. Again, where the Schedule on Page 235 (and the following pages for the other weeks) shows "Cardio Session 1" or "Cardio Session 2" you can use these workouts, if your ability level is 'intermediate'.

Week	Activity	Duration	Intensity
1	Jogging (or cycling, etc.)	2 sessions @ 30 mins	Comfortable pace
2	Jogging (or...your choice of cardio activity)	2 sessions @ 40 mins	Brisk pace, include hills
3	Jogging, running	2 sessions @ 50 mins	Brisk pace, include hills
4	Jogging, running	2 sessions @ 60 mins	Brisk, hilly, include some paced effort, 2 * 5 mins

Strength training workout for **intermediate** level. Once more, where the Schedule on Page 235 (and the following pages) shows "Strength training session 1" or "Strength training session 2" you can use these workouts, if your ability level is 'intermediate'.

Movement	Weight	Repetitions	Notes
Prisoner squats	Hold dumbbells or wear weighted vest	15 to 20	Good form
Push-ups	Bodyweight	20 to 30	Use knees if required
Standing knee raises with hold	Bodyweight	20	Squeeze in abs, engage core
Lunges	Bodyweight	30 each leg	60 total
Shoulder overhead press	Increasing each week	20	Both sides
Shoulder side raise	Increasing each week	20	Both sides
Shoulder front raise	Increasing each week	20	Both sides
Biceps curls	Increasing each week	20	20 each arm
Triceps kickbacks	Increasing each week	20	Reps each arm
Chair dips	Bodyweight, add weight vest if possible	20	Ensure chair stable
Calf raise on step	Bodyweight	20	Hold wall for stability
Standing touch toes	Bodyweight	1 minute	Stretch

Bodyweight HiiT Plan for **intermediate** level.

Movement	Work time	Rest time	Notes
Squats	50 seconds	10 seconds	Holding dumbbells at shoulders
Push-ups	50 seconds	10 seconds	Ideally, no knees
V-Crunches	50 seconds	10 seconds	Caution if you suffer low back pain
Burpees	50 seconds	10 seconds	Full burpees – full!!
Mountain climbers	50 seconds	10 seconds	Non-stop!
Straight lunges	50 seconds	10 seconds	Feel the burn now
Squat thrusts	50 seconds	10 seconds	Old school!
Jump squats	50 seconds	10 seconds	Feeling hard now!

Exercise notes

Strength training routine: You'll feel this is a good step up from the complete beginner level. Always focus on good form, keep the weights manageable. Aim to complete the whole thing in about 15 minutes. Focus on form, not speed. As you get stronger, can you do two circuits? Even three?

Bodyweight HiiT: Now, HiiT is called 'High-Intensity' for a reason. This means that during the 50 seconds of 'work' – you gotta work! I see some folks doing so-called HiiT training (on YouTube) and they are doing a few jumping jacks, popping in 10 push-ups, sitting down to complete a set of 20 sit-ups then grinning at the camera and saying they are all done! The clue is in the name – *high intensity!*

If you try that 8-minute routine above, and you are not red-faced, sweating and puffing and rolling on the floor groaning at the end, you did not try hard enough! Not even close! In this second routine, we've gone to 50 seconds work and 10 seconds rest, just to demonstrate variety. If you struggle with that, try a 40 seconds work, 20 seconds rest version while your fitness builds up.

If you are really short of time, one round will do. But ideally, take two minutes rest and then go around again. Try to build up to doing two, three, even four rounds by Week 4. Anyone for five or six rounds? (Yikes!!)

Advanced workouts

Cardio workout plan for **advanced** trainees.

Week	Activity	Duration	Intensity
1	Running	2 sessions @ 30 mins	Moderate pace
2	Paced running	2 sessions @ 40 mins	Brisk pace, try to find some hills if you can
3	Paced running	2 sessions @ 50 mins	Brisk pace, find some hills if you can, work hard
4	Paced running	2 sessions @ 60 mins	Pace it up, can you run a PB? Can you sprint finish for 500M?

Strength training plan for **advanced** trainees. If you are reading this, then you've set your own level as 'Advanced' so if you know your stuff and are happy with the results you are getting, stick to it. Or, you may like to try a couple of my fitness tests, which I think you'll find offer excellent benefits in terms of all-round strength and muscular endurance.

You could visit the 'Exercise' page on my blog site at mothernaturesdiet.me, and try some of the workouts suggested there. A true classic, **the 6*30 Push-Ups Challenge** is an all-time classic test of muscular endurance and strength.

The **MND Full Body Workload Test** is the original MND test piece (also on the 'Exercise' page on my blog site). Give it a try and let me know (email, Twitter, Facebook, Instagram) how you get on! There are now several variants to the original Workload Test, here you might like to try Variant 2, it's a great workout. You'll need to set your kit up in the gym.

MND Full Body Workload Test: Variant 2

Movement	Weight	Reps	Notes
Push-ups, feet elevated	Bodyweight	30	Feet elevated to create slight decline
Squats	35kg barbell	20	Maintain good form
Pullovers	10kg weight plate	10	Full stretch/ROM
Renegade Rows	8kg or 10kg bells	40	20 each side
Roman Chair sit-ups	10kg	30	Full ROM, hug weight plate to chest
Chin-ups	Bodyweight	10	Good form, no swing
Dips	Bodyweight	20	On parallel bars
Leg raise	Bodyweight	20	On dip bars, allow bent knees
Lunges	Bodyweight	20	Alternating side
Calf raise	Add 20kg	20	On step or box

Rules for this workout:

- No rest between sets
- No rest between circuits
- Finish 3 complete circuits minimum
- Must complete 3 circuits inside 30 minutes
- Advanced: 4 circuits in 40 minutes

If you use a gym with a **Concept II rower**, then you might like to try this excellent strength and fitness test piece.

Rowing	Push-ups
100m	100
200m	90
300m	80
400m	70
500m	60
600m	50
700m	40
800m	30
900m	20
1000m	10

No rest, just switch between indoor rowing on the Concept II and doing push-ups, flipping back and forth between the two as listed. Can you do those push-ups all in one set? The big numbers...70, 80, 90 and 100?

It's a total of 5500 meters of rowing and 550 push-ups, and it hurts. Can you do it in one hour? Now there's a challenge! Time yourself, then aim to get faster, and see how close to an hour you can get it. As an alternative version, you can change push-ups to chin-ups, halve the numbers, and try that version of this workout instead. It's equally tough!

And for the fully advanced trainee, (and it's not strictly strength training, but believe me you need to be strong to complete it) you might like to try the **MND Fitness Workload Test 4**.

Movement	Reps	Notes
3-mile run	3 miles	Fast as possible
Sit-ups or crunches	50	Strict good form
Chin-ups	100	Good form, no swing
Push-ups	150	Good form, full ROM
Mountain climbers	200	Work fast, but maintain good form
Jump rope	250	Any style, fast as possible
2-mile run	3 miles	Fast as possible

It's all bodyweight training, using no additional weight, though the super-advanced trainee may like to try the whole thing wearing a 10kg weight vest for an insanely tough challenge (no thanks!). Work non-stop, moving from one thing to the next. So, you cannot start the chin-ups, until those crunches are done. Then finish **ALL** the chin-ups before starting the push-ups. Your time for this test is from the start of the 3-mile run, to the end of the 2-mile run. Rules:

- Must be non-stop
- Must complete each exercise before moving on to the next
- Time is start-to-finish
- Aim to finish the whole workout in under 80 minutes
- Chin-ups = no swinging/kipping

Bodyweight HiiT Plan for **advanced trainees**. (Hint: this is gonna hurt!)

Movement	Work time	Rest time	Notes
Push-ups	60 seconds	No rest	No rest! No knees!
V-Crunches	60 seconds	No rest	Good form, solid core
Burpees	60 seconds	No rest	Chest-to-floor, full reps
Mountain climbers	60 seconds	No rest	Fast, core locked
Squat thrusts	60 seconds	No rest	Rock 'em out
Plank skiers	60 seconds	No rest	Big firm leaps
Dynamic push-ups with clap	60 seconds	No rest	Get that clap in
Lunge jumping	60 seconds	No rest	Just torture
Sit-ups	60 seconds	No rest	This is an active rest!
Diamond push-ups	60 seconds	No rest	Hit those triceps
Jumping side lunges	60 seconds	No rest	Dynamic movements
Hindu push-ups	60 seconds	No rest	Sorry!
High knees running	60 seconds	No rest	Dynamic, on the spot
T-bar push-ups	60 seconds	No rest	Easy
Jump squats	60 seconds	No rest	Longest 60 secs of your life!

Exercise notes

Bodyweight HiiT for advanced level: Now I am sure you can appreciate, this just got a whole lot harder! 60 seconds per exercise and no rest and straight on to the next movement. That's a 15-minute non-stop HiiT round. Got time? Take 60-90 seconds rest and do it again.

Targets:

- Week 1, start with 2 rounds
- Week 2 = 3 rounds
- Week 3 = 4 rounds (yikes!)
- Week 4 = 5 rounds!! (Rather you than me!)

How to organise your space

Set yourself up for success. We have so many things to deal with, so much to think about and so much change to embrace, the last thing we need is to get 'tripped up' by something simple like stumbling across a bread bin and a toaster during a 'feeling weak moment' or a 'feeling stressed moment'!

Seriously, that happens!

So, **set your kitchen up for success**. It's not 'the law', it's not set in stone, but you might want to do these things (if others in your house agree) to help you stick it through the 28-Day Plan. After that, you won't want to go back!

- Stick the microwave up in the loft – you won't need it
- Ditto the bread bin and the toaster – you won't need those either
- Go through the kitchen cupboards with black bin bags and chuck out everything you don't need that is covered under Core Principle 1, 2, 3 and 4. If it is new and unopened, donate it to a local homeless shelter or charity
- Set up your blender, and/or juicer, near the kettle, in the space the toaster vacated
- Don't have 'that cupboard' full of chocolates, cakes and biscuits. If other people in your house still want that stuff in, ask them if they can stash it in a box somewhere you don't know about it, ask them to help you, it's only 28 days, right?
- Keep the fruit bowl full and easy to reach

Next, **set up your car for success**.

- Empty the sweets and chocolate from the glovebox
- Clean that thing! Valet the car, stop breathing dust, throw sweet wrappers and old coffee cups away
- Keep a pair of jogging shoes or walking boots in the boot, and your packed gym kit bag ready to go – always be prepared

And finally, **set up your workout space for success**.

- Create a space in your home where you are going to do these strength training and HiiT training sessions
- Spare room, garage, corner of the living room? Wherever you plan to work out, set it up ready, put down a yoga mat, **clear distractions** out of arm's reach and out of sight
- Have your dumbbells, hand weights, kettlebells or resistance bands, whatever you need, there, ready, close at hand
- Put up a motivational poster, vision board, some pictures cut from a fitness magazine, or maybe an "at my worst" picture of yourself, ready to be used as your 'before' picture as you work towards your 'after' picture. Put up whatever motivates you to work out
- Timer or stopwatch – have it to hand, all ready to go every day (I use the GymBoss app on my smartphone)
- Plan your jogging routes, be prepared, drive or walk the route first so you know where you are going, if that helps you

Helpful tips and tricks

Karl's Top Tips:

- Don't buy anything advertised as 'low-fat' – it's most likely that it just has a bunch of added sugar instead. Best to buy fresh whole foods, ideally without any label at all. You don't see broccoli or kale in the supermarket with a low-fat label
- Eat a small serving of protein at every meal. Small is palm-sized (that is 2 to 3 eggs, or a chicken thigh or breast, a lamb cutlet, a pork chop, a small tuna or beef steak, these are palm sized. 'Half a cow' is not palm sized!) Protein satisfies so it keeps hunger at bay, and protein nourishes your muscles, helping to combat muscle loss during periods of caloric deficit (when you are trying to lose weight)
- Stop snacking all the time – between meals, in the evening. You don't need it, you will not starve!
- If you must snack, then have an apple, or an orange, or a small handful of almonds
- Stick to the outer aisles in the supermarket. All the fresh whole foods are around the outer edges of a supermarket – they are designed that way (the outer edges are closer to the store rooms for re-stocking shelves.) Those inner aisles are where you'll find the stuff with a longer shelf life, the most processed foods
- Try to create a 12-hour food-free window overnight every night. If you finish your dinner by 7pm in the evening, don't eat breakfast until 7am the next morning. Finish dinner by 8pm, don't eat breakfast until 8am. Can you do that?
- Spread your protein requirements out – eggs, fish, meat, something different at every meal. Personally, I often have eggs for breakfast, fish for lunch and a small serving of chicken or meat in the evening
- Aim to eat fish as often as you eat meat and poultry
- In my opinion, the best fruits are citrus fruits, an apple-a-day and dark, soft, fresh summer berries like blueberries, raspberries and blackberries
- Enjoy free organic food! Plant strawberries in a couple of large pots or trays on your patio or front step. Plant an apple tree in your garden (order one online, get it delivered, less than £50 and it will last decades!) Collect blackberries in autumn

- Alcohol – less is more. Try 28 days teetotal. If you can't do that, then keep your alcohol intake to once per week, perhaps a glass or two on a Friday or Saturday evening. See how it feels, less is more, maybe you'll enjoy it more if it's restricted to a once-per-week treat, part of your Core Principle 12 'allowance'
- Dairy: think quality, not quantity. Enjoy a little organic cheese and yoghurt, shop for quality and animal welfare – organic, free-range, grass-fed
- Base your meals on a palm-sized serving of protein, then fill the rest of the plate with salad or veggies. You can add good fats to your meal to help fill you up, by drizzling good quality extra-virgin olive oil on salads or vegetables, and by adding a knob of grass-fed butter to your veggies
- Try to add nutritious organ meats to a meal when you can. If you are making a family meal like chilli-con-carne or a curry, you can finely dice up some liver and add that in with the minced beef or chicken or pork, and the chances are that no one will notice! I appreciate it's hard to serve up a big liver and bacon casserole and expect fussy kids to tuck in, so hiding liver or kidneys in other meals is a great way to add in the nutrients and the kids will never know!
- If you are constantly stretched for time and you find cooking meals from scratch to be a real challenge, get to love your slow cooker. The slow cooker, or crock pot as it's often called, can be a real time saver. You can load it up with meat and veggies and stock, leave it on 'auto' or 'low' all day, and dinner is ready as soon as you walk in the door, be that 6 hours or 12 hours later, it's always ready when you are
- Get everything you need ready and organised. Set up your kitchen to make life easier (come on, help yourself, it's just 28 days…) and your workout space too

Top Tip: Sunday afternoon 'food prep' time is a big win for a lot of people.

A common challenge many people tell me they face is finding the time to cook meals from scratch during the working week. I'm a busy guy myself and I really do understand this. If I wasn't a home-based worker this would be a huge challenge for me too. The saviour for this problem is 'Sunday afternoon food prep' to get ready for the week ahead!

Roast a joint of ham, or gammon, or a whole chicken, or an oven dish full of chicken drumsticks, thighs and breasts. While this is roasting, stick a big oven dish full of sweet potatoes in your oven too, for just over an hour. Prick the potatoes first, otherwise no prep required, it's super-quick and easy.

Once your joint is done, let it cool a little then carve it all up or slice it all into nice chunky slices, then let everything cool ready for the fridge. Now you have –

- **A bowl of cooked sweet potatoes** to use in the week. You can put one with a salad for a meal, they are tasty cold and you can add a knob of butter or a few squares of feta cheese to add flavour. You can take them to work in a plastic box with salad for lunch
- **A plate full of sliced ham, gammon or chicken** to add to salads and vegetables every day. There's your ham or chicken ready to slice and add to your daily lunch salad. There are slices of gammon to put on your plate in the evening, just add a bunch of steamed, boiled, roasted or stir-fried vegetables

You see, it's not so bad. An hour (tops) on Sunday afternoon and you are all set for the week ahead. It's not too hard, once you get used to it, and preparation is the route to better results. If your life is crazy busy, this is your route forward. I roast a ham joint, some pieces of chicken and some sweet potatoes. Then I make sure I have peppers, carrots, and maybe a pot of hummus, or some kind of home-made salsa dip, and I'm all set for lunches for a busy week ahead.

The 28-Day Plan: Do it twice!

If you do the whole plan twice, that will take you to almost 60 days. Studies show that on average, 66-days is the time it takes for something to become a habit. The difference between an action and a habit, is that the habit no longer requires will power, it's just something you do, it's become your new normal.

Once something is a habit, it's far more likely you will stick with it, for life. For that reason, let's shoot for running through the 28-Day Plan twice. Then it's habit, you've done it, you've nailed this new healthy lifestyle and you're done, your health and your life re-booted for good.

The pages in this **28-Day Plan** tell you **what** to eat, **what not** to eat, what to **shop** for, how to **exercise**, and how **often.** The other 280 pages in this book explain *why*.

This guidance should be enough, it's certainly far clearer and far more concise than anything I had a decade ago to guide me; yet I managed to figure out these steps for myself and lose 101 pounds of unwanted body fat, that's over 7 stones, or 46 kilos of fat. I'm no-one special. If I can do it, you can do it. Ok, you're ready, it's time to get cracking.

Go on then...

...just start.

You can use this page for your own notes.

Three Key Lessons

IMPORTANT LESSONS WE HAVE LEARNED ALONG THE WAY

A t the start, I wrote - while you read this book, as well as introducing you to the *Mother Nature's Diet* healthy lifestyle, I hope to teach you three things.

1. You have a choice. The value of preventive medicine.
2. Eat less, eat better, move more.
3. You are an individual. One size does not fit all, we are all different. Aim for progress, not perfection. Healthy living doesn't need to be hard. You can do it, just start.

You have a choice

In chapter three, 'The *Mother Nature's Diet* Lifestyle', and in chapter six, 'Sidebar: Micronutrients', I explained that *you have more choice over your own health outcomes than most people have been led to believe*. Over the last six or seven years, as I have travelled the country meeting people and delivering seminars and talks, I have consistently found that the majority of the British public do not understand how much control they actually have over their own health.

- We can cut back the starchy carbohydrate and refined sugar in our diet, to (in many cases) almost effortlessly lose unwanted weight
- Vitamins and minerals do a lot more than "good hair and nails" and we can choose to eat a nutrient-dense diet for anti-ageing, better immune function and more energy

- 42% of UK cancer is preventable (that's a Cancer Research UK statistic, I believe the MND lifestyle can take that figure to well over 50%) through making a few simple changes to our diet and lifestyle, and that's all incorporated in *Mother Nature's Diet*
- The MND lifestyle can help you tackle obesity, type-2 diabetes and heart disease/stroke. I believe the majority of cases of these conditions in the UK could be prevented
- The 12 Core Principle address all these issues and more – to give you more choice over your own health outcomes than you knew you had. You can lose weight, feel better, have more energy, resist the signs of ageing, resist ill health, and live a preventive medicine lifestyle to help you (as best as possible) resist chronic degenerative illness as you age

Most people are genuinely unaware they have this choice. Most people I meet assume that heart disease and cancer, ageing badly or feeling sick and tired all the time, are just *inevitable factors of ageing, or bad luck*, and there's not a damn thing they can do about any of it.

Eat less, eat better, move more

Throughout this book I have repeatedly explained the need to eat a little less, and most importantly to eat better.

It's a shift to **fewer calories, more nutrients**.

It's **less food, more nourishment** and that's what many people need.

In the last few decades, car culture has engulfed us, and most people walk less and drive everywhere. Combined with office jobs, online ordering and delivery, and labour-saving gadgets for everything, we are fast becoming a sedentary society [1]. At the same time, the proportion of calories from carbohydrates has been increasing in the nation's diet – people are eating too much 'energy food' but not using enough energy. The end result is an obesity problem.

For some people, 'eat less' is the relevant bit here. It may be that you overeat (and you know it; I meet many people who are very aware that this is their problem) because food is an emotional crutch to you, that's something to work on. Or maybe you need to re-read Core Principle 3, and remove those processed foods from your life that lead to overeating easily-available calories without even feeling particularly full.

Or maybe the 'eat better' bit is relevant to you – perhaps this is where Core Principle 1 will work for you, perhaps you need to remove the bulky starchy carbohydrates from your diet. I meet many people who can easily lose 20 or 30 pounds in a few months just by dumping those starchy carbs, and cutting the refined sugars.

Or perhaps the 'move more' bit is the relevant bit for you. We all need to move, we all need activity and movement in our lives, but some people can tolerate a sedentary lifestyle better than others.

One size does not fit all, we are all different

We are all individuals, we are all different. This theme has come up time and again through this book, you'll see it even right here, above on this very page, as we all have somewhat different needs.

I have explained the flaw in most weight loss diets; they assume a one size fits all approach and that is just not appropriate. I run a 3-day *MND Intensive Workshop* where, among other things, I teach this principle in detail, explaining how you could sit five people down side-by-side to eat the same meal, but they would all derive a different number of calories from that meal, and different amounts of micronutrients, because the people all have different gut flora, genetics, metabolic variations, body size, energy requirements, base metabolic rate, and more.

---

[1] Public Health England: *6 million adults do not do a monthly brisk 10 minute walk.* (2017, Aug 24). Retrieved from
https://www.gov.uk/government/news/6-million-adults-do-not-do-a-monthly-brisk-10-minute-walk

Mother Nature's Diet is different. The 12 Core Principles act as a **broad set of dietary and lifestyle guidelines**, designed to get you moving in the right direction, achieving progress (but rarely perfection) and then as you move forward, you can work on tweaking and adjusting the details to best suit you.

Aim for progress, not perfection, you *can* do it, just start

Just start – that's my advice to you. You can tackle the MND lifestyle in 'one big go' if you are 'a JFDI kinda person', dive in to the 28-Day Plan and follow it to the letter, or you can take it one step at a time. You could work on the 12 CP's in a logical sequence, or you could dip in and out of this book in random order. You could take any one chapter and just work on that, then a day or a week or a month later, work on another. The point is, **just start.** Just do it.

Other key lessons

One of the core themes I have tried to share in this book is that fad diets are largely pointless unless you want fad results.

Lifestyle and consistency

The route to permanent change and lasting results is to adopt a healthy lifestyle. I once heard the brilliant Larry Winget say **"What kind of people go on diets? Fat people. What do healthy people do? They live a healthy lifestyle."** Short and abrupt, perhaps too direct for some people, but oh so true for so many people lost in 'the paralysis of analysis' that is over-thinking diet details.

The reality is that the perfect diet for you, is the diet you stick to. I preach the 90/10 rule, but as we discussed under Core Principle 12, if the 80/20 rule or the 70/30 rule is the best you can stick to long term, then that's what you should do. It's about making progress, not aiming for perfection.

The key focus points of your healthy MND lifestyle should be:

- Consistency: even the most perfect diet in the world is pointless if you can only stick it for a fortnight and then you 'fall off the wagon' and go on a junk food binge! It's what we do consistently, what we do most of the time, the defines our results

- If weight loss is your goal, you need to eat fewer calories than you burn, you need to create a caloric deficit 'most' of the time, so five or six days out of every seven. Eat less, to lose the excess weight you put on over a period of years where you ate more than you needed

- Eat for nutrition, not for fun. Focus on eating for nourishment, rather than using food as an emotional crutch, or a leisure activity

- Ensure you maintain a healthy relationship with food – it is not evil, not a sin, not your friend or enemy, no specific food is particularly 'good' or 'bad', food is just fuel for living your life, and sometimes it's a nice focal point for a social gathering

- If you eat because you are bored, because you are sad, or because you are lonely, recognise that and work on it

- Eat real food – plants and animals. Ensure your diet is based mostly on fresh, nutrient-dense whole foods

- Avoid sugar and processed foods as much as possible, but then when you do enjoy an ice cream on the beach with your kids in summer, or a pizza at your best friend's birthday meal, chill out, enjoy it, don't berate yourself for it and relax knowing that 95% of the time, you are doing everything right. Seriously, the 5% isn't going to kill you

- Keep *excess* starchy carbs out of your diet unless you are very physically active

- Ensure you eat a palm-sized serving of protein at every meal – protein helps maintain your lean mass, your muscles

- Aim for 10-a-day or more, and eat fish several times per week, and try organ meats like liver from time to time. Pack your diet with vitamins and minerals

MND is a lifestyle, not a fad diet, allowing you 10% slack and no calorie counting, but instead putting **good healthy habits in place for life**. Why? Because long term, people do not stick to diets, and that lack of adherence to the protocol (whatever diet they are on) is what causes weight regain. MND is not a diet, it's a lifestyle – you stick with it, and you'll keep the weight off. It's designed to be easy to stick to: no calorie counting; room for a 'treat' now and then; no counting your macros (most regular folks don't even know what their macros are). Get other *exciting things in your life*, and stop using food/alcohol as a distraction/therapy to relieve boredom and make up for what else is missing in your life! MND for life!

You have learned that personal responsibility is the name of the game. All the health advice in this book is simple, but simple does not always mean easy. It's not always going to be easy. There are likely to be tough days. You are going to have to change.

You are going to have to change. If you keep doing what you've been doing, you'll keep getting what you've been getting.

The Sliding Scale

You have learned that skipping your 5-a-day ain't such a smart thing to do! It just might be ageing your prematurely, weakening your immune system, leaving you feeling weak, sick and tired, and making you look pretty crappy for your age!

What can I say? My mum was right – vegetables, liver and fish, they really are good for you!

Personally, I eat about 17-a-day, mostly veggies, probably around 14 servings of vegetables per day, and then two or three servings of fruit per day. For about eight

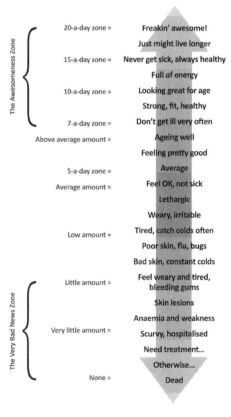

months of the year, I am growing many of those veggies myself, and some of my own fruit. I also eat fish about five times per week, and organ meats probably once-a-week most weeks. I'm packing a nutrient-dense diet and reaping the rewards! How about you? My advice? **Just start.**

Making your life easier

Throughout this book I have tried to give you useful advice for **weight loss, increased energy, resisting the signs of ageing and disease prevention.** In the name of making life easier for you, over the next few pages I just want to pull together the various key points, for each of those topics, that you have learned in this book into some simple lists – a recap by bullet points, you know, to help you out, just in case you forgot to write notes as were reading.

Weight loss tips

Top weight loss tips:

- Stop eating the starchy white 'bloat food', the bread, the cereals, the pasta
- Ditch the sugar, and that includes watching the number of alcoholic drinks you consume, particularly beer
- Ditch the processed, hyperpalatable foods that are sold to hit you at your bliss point, to make you overeat, so you buy more food!
- Develop a daily exercise habit
- Reduce stress – chronic stress contributes to central adiposity (belly fat)
- Activity is your friend. Build a busy, active, fulfilling life, and keep busy every day. Make excuses to move. Leave the lift, take the stairs. Park at the back of the car park
- Don't mistake thirst for hunger! Hunger pangs can often be fought off with a few breaths of fresh air and a glass of water
- Include a palm-sized serving of meat or fish or eggs with every main meal – protein is satiating, it staves off hunger

To have more energy

To have more energy:

- Eat a high nutrient diet
- B vitamins help you make energy, iron helps transport the oxygen around your body to fuel everything that you do, supplying oxygen to working muscles
- You've got to get regular exercise. Exercise improves fitness. It's kind of "more energy makes more energy"
- Make vitamin D from sunshine; 10 minutes a day is better than anything you can get in your diet. Optimal vitamin D aids energy production
- Eat your fish. Eat your green vegetables
- Reduce stress
- Sleep more
- Time outside in Nature

Anti-ageing tips

Top anti-ageing tips:

- Again, eat a high nutrient diet. Eat more vegetables, fish, organ meats, free range eggs, pack in those vitamins and minerals
- Want to have beautiful skin? What will help is vitamins, habitual good hydration, and oxygen from regular aerobic exercise
- Number one longevity tip in the world, develop the habit of going for a walk every day. Move naturally
- Exercise on a daily basis
- Use and retain your muscles and strength to avoid frailty
- Cardiovascular exercise to keep your heart healthy

Immune function and disease prevention

There are two types of disease prevention that we should think about. There is the day-to-day acute illness like coughs, colds and chest infections that we want to resist. Then there are the longer term chronic degenerative diseases, the NCDs that kill 70% of people in our culture – we're talking cancer, heart disease and stroke, type-2 diabetes, COPD and Alzheimer's.

Heart disease and cancer

Here is a sobering dose of reality for you. We're all going to die. There are books and diet plans out there, 'eat to avoid cancer' and 'your diet to stop heart disease' and they're out there saying, "Oh yeah, people have followed this diet and we're *saving lives* around the world."

No diet or exercise plan can *save* lives, we're all going to die. All we can do is *extend* lives.

Fire fighters *save* lives. Paramedics *save* lives. Search and rescue boat crews *save* lives. Seat belts, crash helmets and airbags *save* lives. Diets don't save lives. But what the right diet and lifestyle can do, is **save you from dying young**, save you from dying *prematurely*. The right diet can *extend* your life. My wish for you is that you become one of the people I'm talking about in the future who made it to 98, or 108, not a sad statistic at 58 or 68. **It's not about saving lives, it's about extending them.**

And it's not just about life span, it's about 'healthspan'. I want you to live longer, but not living an unhealthy, unhappy half-life, feeling weak and on heaps of medications. I want you to be full of vitality, living your life fully, busy doing lots with your life and enjoying every moment. We want life to be long, but long and productive, feeling good, enjoying good health, full mobility and plenty of energy.

We want to add years to our life, and life to our years.

In our society, very broadly speaking, one third of people will die from heart disease or stroke, and one third will die from cancer. The remaining third will die from a variety of other causes. **Clearly, finding ways to resist heart disease and cancer for as long as possible is going to form a big part of any 'live longer' strategy.**

Throughout this book I have talked about the benefits of consuming certain nutrients that help your immune system, and talked about the established preventable causes of heart disease and cancer. This is no *pseudoscience nonsense*, no "the truth the doctors aren't telling you" scam rubbish, none of that *quackery* that is so frustratingly prevalent online these days, this is just simple facts that are available from places like Cancer Research UK[2], the World Health Organization[3], the NHS[4], the British Heart Foundation[5] and Public Health England[6]. No nonsense here, just the straight facts, that we could quite easily prevent half of all cancer and heart disease in the UK, extending tens of millions of lives by a decade or more, just by following the advice in this book.

This is the truth. Smoking causes 12% of UK cancer deaths, so don't smoke. Drinking alcohol causes 4% of UK cancer deaths, so don't drink. Being overweight or obese causes around 5% of UK cancers, so maintain a healthy bodyweight. Poor diet contributes around 3% of UK cancers, so eat a better diet - more fruit and veg, a diet higher in nutrient-dense fresh whole foods, and less processed foods and sugar and processed meats. A lack of physical activity causes around 1% of UK cancer deaths, so exercise every day for life.

If you add up the simple diet and lifestyle factors noted in this book, Cancer Research UK suggest that 42% of cancer in the UK could be prevented. As I stated a few pages back, I believe that figure is extremely conservative, and in fact I believe that the lifestyle detailed in this book could prevent at least 50% of the cancer in the UK.

---

[2] *Can cancer be prevented?* (2016). Retrieved from https://www.cancerresearchuk.org/about-cancer/causes-of-cancer/can-cancer-be-prevented
[3] *Prevention of noncommunicable diseases.* Retrieved from https://www.who.int/ncds/prevention/introduction/en/
[4] *Reducing your risk of cancer.* (2016.) Retrieved from https://www.nhs.uk/conditions/cancer/
[5] *Heart and mental health.* Retrieved from https://www.bhf.org.uk/informationsupport/support/health-and-emotional-support/heart-and-mental-health
[6] *Cardiovascular disease: getting serious about prevention.* (2016). Retrieved from https://www.gov.uk/government/publications/cardiovascular-disease-getting-serious-about-prevention

Just let that thought roll around your head for a minute. **At least 50% of the entire cancer burden in the UK. HALF.** Or more. I have collated the relevant tips in this book for you here:

Cancer prevention:

- Don't smoke
- Drink very little alcohol, or quit completely
- Eat a healthy diet
- Veg and fruit: aim for a minimum of 7-a-day, ideally more
- Take regular exercise
- Maintain a healthy BMI
- Enjoy *responsible* sun exposure
- Reduce your exposure to man-made chemicals
- Buy organic, avoid pesticides
- Ensure regular adequate sleep
- Avoid vitamin D deficiency
- Get plenty of sunlight in the day, sleep in a dark room at night

Heart disease prevention:

- Don't smoke
- Maintain a healthy BMI, do not become obese
- Take regular exercise
- Eat a healthy diet
- Eat plenty of omega-3 fatty acids, eat some oily fish weekly
- Maintain a healthy blood pressure
- Quit, or moderate, your alcohol consumption
- **Reduce stress**
- Ensure adequate sleep
- Stay active
- Good hydration
- Be happy, smile, relax

According to the World Health Organisation, and I quote:

"**NCDs account for 63% of all deaths.** Noncommunicable diseases (NCDs), primarily cardiovascular diseases, cancers, chronic respiratory diseases and diabetes, are responsible for 63% of all deaths worldwide."[7]

"**NCDs are largely preventable.** Noncommunicable diseases are preventable through effective interventions that tackle shared risk factors, namely: tobacco use, unhealthy diet, physical inactivity and harmful use of alcohol."[8]

"**Eliminating major risks could prevent most NCDs.** If the major risk factors for noncommunicable diseases were eliminated, at around three-quarters of heart disease, stroke and type 2 diabetes would be prevented; and 40% of cancer would be prevented."[9]

Not my words, the words quoted over above come from the World Health Organisation, the NHS, Public Health England, Cancer Research UK, the British Heart Foundation – these organisations represent the collective intelligence of tens of thousands of people, thousands of scientists, tens of billions of pounds in research budgets, and decades of research.

"Around three-quarters of all heart disease and stroke, three quarters of all type-2 diabetes, and almost half of all cancer, could all be prevented."

---

[7] *NCDs account for 63% of all deaths.* See:
https://www.who.int/features/factfiles/noncommunicable_diseases/facts/en/
[8] *NCDs are largely preventable.* See:
https://www.who.int/features/factfiles/noncommunicable_diseases/facts/en/index4.html
[9] *Eliminating major risks could prevent most NCDs.* See:
https://www.who.int/features/factfiles/noncommunicable_diseases/facts/en/index9.html

Three quarters of all heart disease and stroke, three quarters of all type-2 diabetes, and almost half of all cancer. **Entirely preventable. Completely. Just using the dietary and lifestyle guidance outlined in this book.**

I am sorry, I write and talk very candidly about cancer, please don't think this is blasé or in any way belittling, or that I fail to realise how serious this issue is. The truth is that cancer has affected my life as much as anyone else. I've shed my share of tears. I lost a very good friend of mine, aged just 42, a year after that it was my own mother at 67, three years later we lost my sister-in-law, aged just 47, then the following year another friend only in his early 50s. All cancer. My mother's side of our family all died young, and all mostly to cancer. No one passed age 70. I've spent my share of time sitting bedside, and I've shed my share of tears so I know all about how it feels and cancer affects every one of us and has hurt every family. Everyone's lost someone, cancer is the curse of our times.

But that's partly why this pisses me off so much. I see so many people crying for loved ones, I see so many families hurting, and we're all crying "Why me, why us/him/her... if only they could cure this bastard disease..." and we all go run around the park in a pink skirt, or skydive or night hike in a bra or whatever it is, to raise funds for research – and **that's all very laudable and well intentioned** and I am sure the research is very valuable. But in truth, rather than throwing countless billions at trying to find **a cure**, if we all just ate a better diet, drank less booze, quit smoking, got some exercise and made a few other small changes, half of this entire disease burden would be gone in a single generation. We need to follow the advice in this book, and focus on **prevention** first and foremost. *Prevention is better than cure.*

If someone came up with a magic pill tomorrow that could 'cure cancer' and they gave it to millions of people and 50% of those people were cured – that person would immediately be given a Nobel Prize, and would no doubt quickly become a billionaire and the toast of the scientific and pharmaceutical world. Yet, here we have the WHO, the NHS, PHE, CRUK and the BHF telling folks how to stop 50% of cancer happening in the first place, **and most people can't be bothered to put down their wine and cake long enough to read the ***king advice. Yes, this really pisses me off.**

We need to teach our children to reframe how they think about these diseases. We need to change the language used around heart disease and cancer.

You don't 'get' cancer – you grow it. You don't 'get' heart disease – you develop it.

Cancer isn't contagious (OK, maybe some 5% or 10% of cancers start from a virus or infectious agent) you don't 'get' cancer by touching someone with cancer or breathing cancerous air. You don't catch it. You grow it, and the dietary and lifestyle **choices** you make play a major role in creating an 'inner environment' in your body, which will either encourage or discourage that growth.

Heart disease isn't 'an event' that happens in a moment, like a car accident. You don't get it, you grow it, you *develop* it, over a long period of time, **it's a process, not an event.** Your lifestyle choices and your nutrition choices can either encourage or discourage that process. Cancer and heart disease, the global top two killers. **You have more choice than you know.**

Save the NHS while we are at it

I have mentioned the NHS many times in the pages of this book. Personally, I think it is an amazing and best-in-the-world health service, and I think we are very lucky in the UK to have our NHS, and we should all work hard as a nation to resist privatisation. If people are not motivated to look after themselves now, privatised healthcare will be an extremely uncomfortable push towards better personal responsibility. Private healthcare is expensive, very expensive, and it will hit and hurt families on lower incomes far more than the wealthy. Wise up now Britain – save the NHS now or you'll pay a high price when it's gone.

Two of the biggest areas of cost that the NHS has to deal with are funding drugs and funding hospitals. The burden of dealing with cancer and heart disease are 'front and centre' in both these areas of cost. Add on obesity-related ill health and the fast-growing cost of treating type-2 diabetes and diabetes complications, and we are looking at tens of billions per annum in costs.

Look back over the last few pages – three quarters of heart disease and type-2 diabetes and half of all cancer is entirely preventable. If we want to save the NHS, the best way to do it is to follow the healthy living guidelines in this book. Let's just stop the heavy disease burden in the first place, stop getting sick in the first place, and we can save the NHS tens of billions every year.

Less cancer, less heart disease, less suffering, less misery, less of our tax payer's money handed over to giant pharmaceutical companies, help keep taxes lower and ensure nurses and doctors are paid fairly and don't have to work such excessive hours. It's entirely possible, and it's simple stuff, it's all outlined in this book. No rocket science, just simple and enjoyable healthy living.

I think far too many people have this stupid mentality that they can just live how they like, do anything, bask in hedonism, make no effort to look after themselves, 'break' themselves through partying and laziness, and the NHS will fix them up 'when it all goes Pete Tong'. People think they can just drink and smoke and do whatever they like, ignore advice to eat 5-a-day or take regular exercise, knowing they will end up in poor shape, and it's their 'right' to do that, because they have paid their taxes, they have paid for an NHS to look after them when things go wrong.

That just shows a total lack of personal responsibility. This is not just my own observation, I have spoken to nurses who say this, doctors who say this same thing, and I have met those members of the public who live this way and admit this too. It's wrong, it's flawed thinking, it won't last forever. Wake the hell up.

One nurse I spoke to in a hospital, stood beside several million pounds' worth of scanning machinery, said "The trouble is, we have become extremely good at fixing things, at keeping people alive, and the public know it, and expect it. They just go out and wreck themselves, then come to us to be fixed. We can fix them, but all this stuff costs an absolute fortune, and no one wants to increase their taxes to pay the bill. Well, we can't have it both ways. It won't last, it can't last."

I look around our great nation and I see so many people who are sleep deprived; stressed out (often over money and material possessions); 75% of the population are vitamin D deficient; 73% eating less than the 5-a-day vegetables and fruits that are recommended as part of a healthy diet; two thirds of the nation don't exercise enough; a quarter of all adults drink more than the recommended limit; most people are consuming too much sugar and processed foods; 90% or more of people don't buy organic so they are likely consuming pesticide residues year after year; two thirds of folks don't eat enough fresh fish; most people don't get enough fresh air or drink enough clean water; folks are filling their homes with sprays, putting chemicals on their skin; one third of the nation are obese, one third are overweight; too many people living sedentary lives, a quarter of all adults take no exercise at all. This is all bad news.

It all adds up. The risk factors stack up.

These diseases (these NCDs, heart disease, type-2 diabetes, many cancers) are what is called *multifactorial*, in other words it's rarely one single cause, but a number of causal factors that stack up, multiplying the odds you will develop heart disease or cancer. Everyone likes to blame obesity on their genes, diabetes on bad luck "well I just followed the diet recommended by doctors, it's not my fault", they think heart disease is some kind of lottery and cancer just comes with ageing.

But you know differently, you've learned in this book, you now know: **You have a choice.**

An analogy

- An apple a day
- Regular daily exercise
- Don't smoke

People know these things are good for us, this is pretty universally recognised common sense health advice. But what if you skip the apple a day, and have three chocolate biscuits per day instead?

Would that work? How long could you get away with that before life taught you the error of your ways? Science aside, you know as well as I do, you just know that in time, you'd learn why the saying is "an apple a day" and not "three chocolate biscuits a day". Right? You have to be smarter than that. I have an analogy for you, coming up, to help illustrate this.

People like to think that their behaviour is "not that much of a big deal" because they do not suffer the ill effects immediately. There is a **long time-lag** between **cause** and **effect**.

For example, in the UK, it's a serious worry that a lot of children are eating far too much sugar. Recent surveys suggest that on average, children in the UK are eating more than twice the recommended maximum amount of added sugar. It's not that many parents are feeding their kids five chocolate bars per day. In reality, it's largely because of the amount of sugar in soft drinks and fizzy drinks, and all the sugar added to processed foods. As you have read in this book, from sliced bread to pizza, from crispy snacks and breakfast cereal, to milk drinks and tomato ketchup, everything has a ton of added sugar.

These kids are eating more than twice as much sugar as is recommended, day in day out, year in year out. But most parents pretty much shrug it off and look at their kids and say "Well, he ate that stuff yesterday, and the day before, and last week and the week before, last month and the month before, and look at him, he looks fine, no worries." And "Leave them alone, they're just kids, stop being 'the food police', let them live a little, let them enjoy dessert now and then, you did when you were a kid."

True, I did enjoy dessert now and then when I was a kid. The difference is, when I was a kid, there wasn't all the sugar added to processed foods, we rarely drank fizzy drinks, and we grew up with fewer cars, TVs, tablet computers, games consoles and social media. We played outside because there wasn't so much else to do.

This issue is real. In the UK now, one quarter of 5-year-olds are either overweight or obese. One third of 11-year-olds. And it's increasing every decade.

Metabolic damage builds over a long time

And what few parents realise is that all that sugar is causing metabolic damage. Science is slowly showing us that metabolic dysfunction is a root cause in far more than just type-2 diabetes. Metabolic syndrome is now identified as a major causal factor for obesity, for heart disease and stroke, it is rapidly being implicated in many forms of cancer, there is a movement to see Alzheimer's Disease renamed as 'type-3 diabetes', and metabolic syndrome is additionally being looked at in relation to autoimmune diseases, dementia, arthritic conditions and more.

Healthy metabolic function, and good insulin sensitivity, are regulated by several mechanisms. Sugar in the diet is one factor, so is exercise, stress and gut flora. All are potential problem areas in our **processed food crazed, sedentary society.**

If these young kids are eating twice as much sugar as they should, from age three or four on upwards, and lacking exercise too...we may find in years to come, that metabolic dysfunction, primarily insulin resistance, starts rearing its ugly head many years earlier in these people's adult lives. Instead of a type-2 diabetes epidemic hitting people in their 40s and 50s, we may start seeing it hitting large numbers of people in their 30s. Heart disease in the 50s and 60s, might become heart disease in people in their 40s.

Here comes that analogy

Imagine you are young again! Just 22 years of age. And you have a stash of cash, say one hundred thousand pounds, perhaps you won on the lottery, and you decided to take your hundred grand in cash, and keep it in a big box in the corner of your living room. Day one you are going to **feel** pretty loaded! 'Yay, I've got a hundred grand in ten-pound notes in my living room! Happy days! I'm rich! I *feel* rich!'

You take a grand the first month and blow it having a good time...meals out, you rent a sports car for a weekend, you stay in a couple of nice hotels, you visit a couple of expensive bars. A grand soon goes. The next month, same again. It's cool, you've been partying it up for two months and look, you still have £98 grand in cool hard cash, the world is good! Party on!

You go all year. That was £12 grand, one each month. Yeah but look it's barely made a dent in the pile, you still have a massive heap of £88 grand sitting there, and it **looks** good, and you are having a ball. So, you go another year. And another.

It's all so much fun.

After eight years and four months, you go to the box to get 'this month's fun money' out and "Oh shit, WTF, the box is empty...where did all my money go?" Now, you don't feel so rich any more. **Now you feel broke.** You feel sad. The fun is over.

You won the lottery when you were 22, you were loaded, you thought you had it all, you were set for life, you had a hundred grand. Now you're 30 and broke, all you have left to show for it is a speeding ticket and a hangover. (Yeah, I know, you had some good times along the way...)

My old mum always used to say "A fool and his money are soon parted." Indeed, my mum was right.

Now, alternative scenario: the smart 22-year-old might have invested that £100 grand in a small rental property, and then enjoyed a modest income from that property of, say, for example, £400 per month, for ever, for life, which at 22, might be another 80 years.

What would you rather have from age 22 - £1000 per month for eight years and four months, or £400 per month for your entire life, slowly going up with inflation as you age? And you still have your capital, growing, working for you, invested in the property market.

Of course, anyone with a brain can see that investing the money into property would have been a much, much smarter thing to do. Because that money, as a pot of cash, **if we just keep digging in and taking out**, and we never add capital back into the pot, we never invest, **then the pot will slowly deplete.**

And so it is with your metabolic health.

Yes, you can eat two or three times the recommended guideline amount of sugar today and wake up just fine tomorrow, but you have to understand that if you keep doing it **every day**, month after month, year after year, just like that young person dipping in to that pot of cash, you are slowly depleting the reserves, and not putting anything back in.

When the pot runs dry, when your bodily tissues become insulin resistant, when your pancreas can no longer produce enough insulin when it needs it, you've just hit personal ground zero. You took it all out, and now there's nothing left. You're broke. You're broken. You're all done.

You've got to be smarter than that.

If you have a child, or spouse, or friend, (or you?) who is consuming a lot of sugar but not obese, don't be naïve enough to think that it's all fine, the sugar isn't doing them any harm. It is. **It's likely still damaging their metabolic health.**[10] Slim people can develop metabolic syndrome too.[11] Slim people can

---

[10] Bradshaw, P. T., Monda, K. L., & Stevens, J. (2013). Metabolic syndrome in healthy obese, overweight, and normal weight individuals: the Atherosclerosis Risk in Communities Study. *Obesity (Silver Spring, Md.), 21*(1), 203–209. doi:10.1002/oby.20248

[11] Spencer, E. A., Pirie, K. L., et al., (2008). Diabetes and modifiable risk factors for cardiovascular disease: the prospective Million Women Study. *European Journal of Epidemiology, 2008; 23*(12): 793-9. doi: 10.1007/s10654-008-9298-3

develop insulin resistance too.[12] Slim people get diabetes too. Slim people get heart disease too. Slim people get cancer too. **Slim people die too.**

- Stop being dumb
- An apple a day keeps the doctor away
- A daily exercise habit keeps you fit
- Saving and investing a little of your income sets you in good stead for old age
- Saving and investing in your health will ensure you reach that old age
- Wise up
- Don't die of ignorance or stupidity

My invitation to you is to…

"Take your health seriously, before something serious takes your health."

---

[12] Devaraj, S., & Jialal, I. (2016). The skinny on metabolic syndrome in adolescents. *Translational pediatrics, 5*(2), 97–99. doi:10.21037/tp.2016.03.06

Frequently Asked Questions

A FEW ANSWERS TO THE QUESTIONS I ANSWER MOST OFTEN

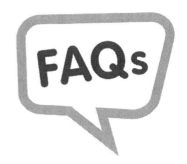

This isn't an exhaustive list, I think that with almost 300 pages behind us already, we really want to keep this pretty brief so you can crack on with your new healthy lifestyle.

Some of the most common questions I get asked about the MND lifestyle are:

- What about legumes?
- Coffee: good or bad?
- Is MND anything to do with Motor Neurone Disease?
- What oil should I cook with?
- Do I have to go teetotal?

And there are several more. These are all addressed online, please just visit the FAQs page on my blog site[1], and you can find all of these popular questions answered there.

What's the point in all this healthy living? I might get run over by a bus tomorrow!

You might, but it's unlikely. According to data from the Office of National Statistics, in 2009 the total number of people in the UK who died from being run over by a bus (or lorry) was 79. In the same year, 160,000 died from heart disease and 140,000 died from cancer. 644 died from falling down a flight of stairs, 93 people died from falling off a building and 18 people drowned in their own bath.

So, if you want to live longer, don't leave your fate to the buses. Instead, follow *Mother Nature's Diet* to prevent heart disease and cancer, be careful on the stairs and take a shower instead of a bath.

---

[1] Please visit *Mother Nature's Diet* blog at
https://mothernaturesdiet.me/faqs/

The whole "do calories matter?" debate. Well, do they matter?

If carbs are the most argued-over topic in nutrition today, then 'whether or not calories matter' comes in a close second.

Let me just nail it in simple terms, as once again this topic warrants a whole book on its own, so it's a rabbit hole we don't want to go too far down right here and now.

- If you are looking at weight management from what we might call "the 50,000 ft view" then calories do matter. **Broadly** speaking, for the majority of people in our **society** who are overweight or obese, the simple truth remains that they eat too much, they eat too much of the wrong things (mainly talking sugar and carbs and highly processed foods here folks) and they don't move enough. That is, they are living broadly inactive lives and yet eating a diet that packs in a lot of energy from readily usable calories which they are just not using. For the most part, they are in caloric excess

- When we screw down to the close-up view, i.e. when we start looking at small groups and **individuals**, picking case examples, and looking at the nuances of an individual's diet, at a specific point in time, then measuring calories becomes pretty much pointless. That is to say, the whole equation of "if you eat 3500 less calories this week, you'll be a pound lighter by next week – and it's all body fat you are losing" is mostly nonsense

- **Eat less, eat better and move more**, is great advice for *whole populations* that are seeing a rising obesity trend. But if you start looking at *individual* 'person X' in specific 'time-period Y' then counting calories becomes ineffective because of the dozens of other variables and factors at play, and as no one size fits all, for every person the combination of all those factors in different

 Can't I have oats for breakfast?

You have a choice. I have shared what I have learned with you in this book, but I'm not there in your kitchen every morning to fix your breakfast for you. It's down to you now.

Someone always asks me…

- "If I do most of what you say, can I have oats for breakfast?"
- Or… "Can I have quinoa for lunch?"

- "How about couscous for dinner?"
- "Are roast potatoes allowed?"
- "Can I just eat bread at the weekends?"
- "Can I have a glass of red wine every day? That's what the French do? Isn't it?"
- "But I don't really like green veg..."
- "I hate fish..."
- "Liver? Yuk! No way!"
- "Can I be good Monday-to-Friday and then eat what I like at the weekends?"

You have a choice. I have told you what I know, and I have explained that Core Principle 12 is open to flexibility and your interpretation. At the end of the day, **your perfect diet is the one you stick to**, the one that becomes a permanent lifestyle, not a fad.

So, ask yourself, how *much*, and how *quickly*, do you want the *results*? How much do you want it? **You decide. You have a choice.**

 ### Cholesterol: Should I worry?

It seems that for my entire adult life, the experts have been telling us that high cholesterol is a major health concern, and leads to heart disease, the number one killer worldwide. This has become such a big deal that over the last few decades the recommended acceptable high level of cholesterol has been brought down and down, and some are recommending it comes down lower still. Doctors have already put millions of people in the UK on statin drugs to lower their cholesterol. If the upper limit of cholesterol comes down any lower, an overwhelming majority of UK adults and many children will be considered eligible to take statins – for life – at a cost of untold billions to the NHS.

Gosh, it makes you wonder how anatomically modern man ever got through 185,000 years without statins. (Ummm...maybe our diet was different back then...?) And no, 'caveman' didn't die at 35.[2]

I am not a doctor, I am not medically qualified in any way, I don't even have a degree in human biology, so I am not in any way qualified to advise you on what your cholesterol level should be, or whether or not you should

---

[2] See my blog: *Myth busting – Part 9.*
https://mothernaturesdiet.me/2016/05/05/myth-busting-part-9/

take a statin drug. It would be unethical, irresponsible and unprofessional of me to attempt to give you, my unknown reader, any kind of one-size-fits-all medical advice. I recommend you talk to your doctor about that.

With that repeated disclaimer in mind, now I will share my *personal opinion*, after years of reading on this topic. Over the last decade I have met a boat-load of people who take a statin every day, and yet they have never had a heart attack, they do not suffer from painful angina, and they actually display no symptoms at all of any ill health. No obvious obesity, high blood pressure or any such thing. Yet they have a cholesterol reading slightly over 5.0mmol/L, they are over 50, they perhaps are 20 pounds overweight, and they may have blood pressure slightly higher than bang-on average, and for this, statins are prescribed. I find this odd. Why would anyone take a drug, for life, that has known side-effects, some serious, when they have no symptoms of ill health and the evidence that these drugs work in primary prevention is scant at best?

Let's take a quick (and honestly incomplete) look at what cholesterol does in a human body.

Cholesterol is an incredibly important compound and without any, you would be dead. Cholesterol is the molecule that your body uses to manufacture steroid hormones, most notably the sex hormones, oestrogen, progesterone and testosterone. Your stress hormones, such as cortisol, are also made from cholesterol.

Cholesterol and sex hormones

If a woman can't make enough oestrogen and/or progesterone, her monthly cycle will fail, she will not be able to conceive.

If a man can't make enough testosterone, his sperm count will fall until he can no longer produce enough sperm to ensure impregnating a female.

Therefore, if men and women all had really, really low cholesterol, we could not conceive and make babies, and **the human race would die out.**

Cholesterol plays an essential role in maintaining cell integrity, in **all** cells in **all** animals (including humans), by helping to form the membrane structure of the cells.

Therefore, if we had no cholesterol, **all humans** and all other animals on Earth for that matter, **could not exist**. 100 trillion cells in a human being, cholesterol is an essential part of every single cell. Interesting.

If a pregnant woman takes a statin, she is very likely to give birth to a baby with massive and severe **birth defects**. This is because the statin reduces cholesterol production which badly affects her foetus, and proper brain development, limb and facial structure, among other things, is impaired. In the drug leaflet in the box, all statins warn against use in pregnancy. That highlights how important cholesterol is for 'making new human beings' as it is one of the fundamental substances that is required in large amounts.

Humans synthesize **vitamin D** (itself a steroid hormone responsible for activation of almost 5% of the protein-encoding genes in the human genome) from cholesterol. Without adequate vitamin D we cannot form strong bones and teeth properly, and children would suffer from major developmental problems.

A normal healthy human will produce about 90% of his or her vitamin D needs (depending on age, skin tone, climate, genetics, and more) from cholesterol, just from regular daily sun exposure from normal living.

Most of the cholesterol we need, **we make ourselves**. Again, typically, for the average person, a human will make about 80% of their cholesterol needs every day, and then look for the last 20% to come from diet. But cholesterol is **so important** that we cannot live without it, *so if your diet provides less, your body just makes more to compensate.*

Let's just be clear:

- Cholesterol is essential to make sex hormones, without which, the human race would stop reproducing and die out
- Cholesterol is so important in a growing foetus, that if the cholesterol supply from the mother to her foetus is interrupted, the baby will likely be born with serious birth defects
- Cholesterol is present, and essential, in every cell in our bodies, and has been for millions of years of evolution
- Cholesterol is essential for vitamin D production, to help us grow healthy strong bones and teeth
- Cholesterol is so important, that our bodies make most of what they need every day, and if we don't eat enough in our diet, the body will just make more to compensate

And this stuff is supposed to be killing us. WTF?

Really? A billion years to evolve life on Earth and you came up with that design, Mother Nature? WTF, Are you for real? Was this some kind of evolutionary mistake?

I don't think so.

Personally, I follow the work of THINCS, The International Network of Cholesterol Sceptics[3], and in particular I avidly follow the blog of Dr Malcolm Kendrick[4], as he continues his life's work investigating the true causes of heart disease. I would encourage you to keep an open mind about cholesterol, and talk to your doctor about following a healthy lifestyle like *Mother Nature's Diet* as an alternative to taking statins.

Worldwide, making statins is **a $30 billion-dollar business**. That's worth remembering.[5]

Personally, my own total cholesterol reading varies between 5.1 and 5.4mmol/L, over the last few years, and I'm in the best health of my life. According to government guidelines, this is a tad high! I think that's nonsense, but that's my personal opinion. Of course, I have built all the heart-disease-preventing knowledge I can into *Mother Nature's Diet*, and I firmly believe that MND makes for an excellent preventive-medicine lifestyle.

FAQs   **MND, is it part of the low-carb trend?**

Mother Nature's Diet is not a strict low-carb diet as has become very popular in recent years. While there is no doubt that low-carb and ketogenic diets have proven to be extremely beneficial for some people, that is not what we are advocating here. In fact, this is a great example of the fact that 'one size does not fit all' and a great example of the 'beware of prescriptive diets' point.

I recommend that "most normal" people quit grains and starchy carbs, but athletes will need to eat more starchy carbs than everyone else. That doesn't mean athletes should eat a load of white bread and cereals...just eat **good** healthy natural starchy carbs, such as sweet potatoes, squash, pumpkin,

---

[3] Learn more: http://www.thincs.org/

[4] See: https://drmalcolmkendrick.org/

[5] *Statins: the drug firms' goldmine.* (2011) The Telegraph from https://www.telegraph.co.uk/news/health/news/8267876/Statins-the-drug-firms-goldmine.html

parsnips and carrots. Remember, one size does not fit all. I tend to say MND is a 'healthy carbs diet' rather than a low-carb diet.

Non-athletes, most folks who are in their 40s and 50s, who do not exercise more than a few hours per week, who are overweight, will find that eating lots of starchy carbs can hamper weight loss efforts (as detailed in Core Principle 1). But the small percentage of our society who are athletes will likely want more of those starchy carbs in order to maintain optimal performance. Bodybuilders and strength athletes will need carbs post-workout to refuel muscles for growth, and endurance athletes might find that starchy carbs in their diet help them to avoid feeling burned out and exhausted. (Personally, as a marathon runner, my performance improved when I switched to low carb.)

There is no one solution for all people!

And this is all a good example of why MND is not a prescriptive 'low carb' diet. Low carb is 'all the rage' these days, but we do not promote low carb specifically. Living the MND way, carbs are on the menu every day – vegetables and fruits are natural carbs. We eat vegetables at pretty much every meal, and fruits in moderation. Beware of health advice that is completely restrictive, such as 'don't eat carbs' as this is a sign of nutrition advice that is trying to apply 'one size fits all' mentality.

Low-carb living is a great place to start for weight loss goals. Hobby athletes engaging in moderate levels of moderate-intensity exercise, in my opinion, can often thrive on a low-carb diet (it works for me). Athletes working at high volume or high intensity, will almost certainly need higher amounts of carbs. There is no one answer, nutrition for athletic performance is a wonderfully complex topic, and I would recommend you hire a knowledgeable trainer to help you set up the optimal training and nutrition plan for you.

FAQs

Isn't a healthy lifestyle really boring? No smoking? No cakes? No alcohol? No drugs? No fun?

No, not boring, *just different*. It may feel 'awkward' at first. If all your friends eat junk food for dinner every night, and if your entire social life revolved around the local pub, then it may feel difficult. For me personally, that first year off alcohol was awkward…I kept trying to still socialise in the old ways, but with me being the odd one out, the only sober one. That was quite hard.

Eventually, things moved on.

In time, you find a new way:

- Different foods
- Different social activities
- Different friends
- Different interests
- Different fun

Now, instead of Saturday nights with my drinking buddies, it's Sunday mornings with my running or cycling buddies. Instead of meeting friends for a few drinks and a curry, it's meeting friends for a Sunday dog walk and pub lunch. Instead of meeting a mate in the pub for a catch up, it's a coffee shop.

I meet friends and we go walking, cycling or running for a catch up and chat, and a coffee afterwards. It's the same friends, just a change of setting. Still happy, still laughter, still good times, just that you feel better and live longer. I have just as many friends, socialise just as often, laugh just as often, and enjoy life. The difference is I am sober, 101 pounds lighter, I don't feel like crap with a hangover the next day and I hope I'll live for an extra 20 or 30 years more. **Not boring, just different.**

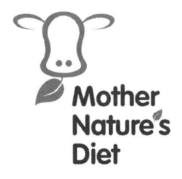

Why have you not provided loads of references to research papers to support every Core Principle and the claims you make about food and nutrition?

Throughout this book I have largely, and entirely purposefully, avoided getting into any kind of detailed discussions on specific scientific details such as the saturated fat versus polyunsaturated fat debate, the low-carb versus high-carb debate, the 'calories do matter' versus 'calories don't matter' debate, and many more contentious issues besides.

You will also surely have noticed that I have tried to keep the references and footnotes to a minimum - not *too many* of those tiny little superscript numbers throughout the text, leading you to 47 pages of detailed references at the back of the book.

All with good reason!

I shall explain in a few simple (but lengthy) statements, why I do not offer an extensive section of scientific references to **support every Core Principle** and every statement in this book, and why I think that in fact this book is better off without them. You will have seen a few references at the bottom of the pages as you have read the book, but hopefully not too many. I have generally included them for the things that might seem less like hard science, and more like "open to interpretation". This includes sections of the book such as the **'Sidebar: Micronutrients'** chapter, which tackles "Karl science" and not any widely accepted or proven theory, so I have included a few references there to help you understand my way of thinking, should you wish to read a little more.

Then in **Core Principle 3**, I included some references to further reading to back up what I have written around the subject of manufacturers making foods these days that lead us to overeat, even after we have eaten what we actually need. And in **Core Principle 4**, I provide some references to read more about the possible harmful effects of chemicals in our food, on our skin, in the air we breathe and in our homes; and in **Core Principle 11** I have included references to substantiate the potentially 'hippie tree hugging woo woo science' idea that time spent in nature is good for us in real, measurable, biological ways.

But I have not provided extensive references to research papers for each and every Core Principle, particularly around all matters pertaining to food, nutrition and disease prevention. There are **four main reasons** for this, please allow me to explain those reasons.

Reason 1) Remember 'My Story' - I read 847 of those books and the papers they refer to, and frankly, I ended up more confused and more uncertain than before I started. I'm not a PhD, I don't have a degree in molecular biology, I'm just a regular guy who doesn't wanna die at 64 of colon cancer. I'm not the smartest guy on the planet, but nor am I stupid. I can read and understand published research, I can check references, I can look for conflicts of interest and I can check and understand research methodologies. Before writing *Mother Nature's Diet*, I worked in research (in the telecoms industry) for 19 years.

Yet, for all my learning and researching health, nutrition, diet, fitness and disease, when all the science was studied and done, it left me utterly confused. I find that in truth, for pretty much **any** of the hotly contested topics in the world of diet and disease, if you care to look, you can find a dozen papers of seemingly good quality that **support both sides of any argument**, and another two dozen in the middle concluding that 'further research is required'. We are left unconvinced. Those who wish to support one view, can cherry pick and quote accordingly, and those who wish to rebuke them, can cherry pick from the other side. I see this in virtually every argument, in almost every press piece, blog, and book review.

Over the last decade, I have found this to be the case for the causes of heart disease, associations between dairy milk and breast cancer, high carb or low carb, saturated fat versus polyunsaturated fat, is cholesterol good for you or bad for you, HiiT training versus steady state cardio, whether or not 'eat less and move more' is relevant and useful advice, and a dozen further topics besides.

Reason 2) Based on what people tell me, the lay reader generally does not want to wade through 38 pages of references – it's downright off-putting to many people. I have been told by many people looking for simple advice on how to lose weight and feel better, than if they pick up a book and see pages upon pages of references at the back, they disregard it, because it's off-putting to think that you need a science degree to try to understand it. In this regard, I have tried to make this book self-explanatory, based on common sense, trial and error, and my own life experience.

In all honesty, I really don't think the reader should have to go off and read a hundred or more research papers in order to make sense of what is written in this book. The book should be, broadly speaking, wholly-contained and self-explanatory. The people who follow me and my work in *Mother Nature's Diet*, the people who join our membership programs and come to our live seminars, trust me that I have read all those books and checked all those references for them, and what I present is the summary and distillation of what I learned along the way. This is the service I offer, it's my value add.

People who have already read this book, and adopted the 12 Core Principles as a sustainable healthy lifestyle, tell me that one of the things they like about this book, is that it bridges the gap between the heavyweight scientific books, and the 'fad diet' books that fail to reference any research in support of their claims. As one reader said "It's the missing link between academic books and commercial ones."

Reason 3) Frankly, this book doesn't make any wild claims or postulate any scientific theories that might need extensive references to back them up. Probably the **most outlandish and potentially contentious** things claimed in this book are as follows:

- Most of us should cut back on our consumption of **grains and starchy carbs** (Core Principle 1). I explain that this is for several reasons, but the main two are that people are just not as active these days as they used to be, and just don't need 30% to 50% of their diet to be based on 'slow release energy' foods. (More on this, with references, in the coming pages.) The second reason is that if you switch out those bulky carbs for more salads and vegetables, you'll be eating a lower-calorie, higher-nutrient-density diet. It's pretty simple stuff, and pretty irrefutable. It's true, it's common sense and it works

- **Added sugar** in our diet is a problem (Core Principle 2), contributing to both weight gain across the population of the UK and type-2 diabetes, and by definition, the antinutrient properties of refined sugar could, technically, see it classified as a mild poison. To be clear about this word "antinutrient", there are many foods that contain antinutrient compounds. Phytic acid, enzyme inhibitors, amylase inhibitors, chelating agents, goitrogens, lectins, protease inhibitors, and tannins are all compounds found in plants, grains and legumes, and all have antinutrient properties. Such compounds are common in some of the plants we love to hail as super healthy, such as cruciferous vegetables like cabbage, kale and broccoli. The key difference is, eating these plants offers many other beneficial compounds, such as fibre and many micronutrients (minerals), whereas eating refined sugar offers nothing but insulin-spiking, obesity-promoting calories, which come with an antinutrient effect

- Sugar (CP2) and highly processed foods (CP3) are **somewhat addictive**. It's true, they are, food manufacturers go to great lengths and great expense to make these hyperpalatable foods so desirable that *you eat more than you need*, and then go back and buy more[6]. In my book, that counts as "addictive" even if the mechanism is more one of habit than biology. Hyperpalatable foods are delicious, they lead to overeating, they create a type of 'food addiction' that is contributing to obesity. That's an ugly truth, sorry

Apart from those three things, I really don't think this book raises any issues that anyone will find debatable or contentious. And if anyone is tempted to say, of those three factors, "Well, you can't say they apply to everyone, you can't just give that blanket advice to all people..." – Nope, you are quite right, I can't. Maybe you noticed, **a couple times**, reading this book, that I mention the idea that *one size does not fit all*, and we should try these things out and see if we get positive improvements in our health as a result.

Of course, a cynic might say something like "Oh now he's just sitting on the fence. He doesn't cast his lot in with the Registered Dietitians teaching The Eatwell Guide, and he's scared to go all-in with the LCHF camp telling everyone to eat a diet high in saturated fat. He won't go one way or the other, because he's not done the research. He's not an academic, not a researcher, not a medical doctor, he's sitting on the fence."

Nope, that's not it. I could quote for you a dozen academics, researchers and medical doctors for both camps, I have read all their research, and I think they are all missing one point.

One size does not fit all!!!

I don't recommend anyone specifically eats a diet high in saturated fat, and I don't recommend anyone specifically eats a diet high in starchy carbs. Because, when was the last time anyone went into a British supermarket and saw a sign hanging over an aisle saying "This aisle: saturated fat" or "This aisle: starchy carbohydrates"?

Never.

People don't eat macronutrients, **they eat food**, and that's generally either *fresh whole foods*, or *packaged processed foods*. I recommend people eat a diet largely made up of the former, and let their saturated fats and starchy carbs fall into place from there.

---

[6] Reading for further interest on this fascinating topic: *The Extraordinary Science of Addictive Junk Food.* New York Times Magazine. (2013, Feb 20). Retrieved from https://www.nytimes.com/2013/02/24/magazine/the-extraordinary-science-of-junk-food.html

Reason 4) [And this one might rattle a few cages.] Frustratingly, a considerable proportion of published research looking at aspects of diet, nutrition and disease, is fundamentally flawed in one way or another. This is a genuine headache for everyone – from researchers, to journal editors, to policy makers and the general public.

Research may be biased due to a **conflict of interests**, such as funding by a drug company, or research may be unreliable due to **poor research methodologies** or poor study design. These issues are very real.

Just looking at the ethics of pharmaceutical companies, as one possible way that published research is biased, it becomes clear that we should exercise some concern. I once got into an argument with a lovely friend about drug companies and their unethical business practises. Sadly, I lost that friend over the argument, which is a real shame. I have no axe to grind personally with any of the big drug companies, or the industry as a whole, but I do think this is an important issue because a large percentage of all research labs and research departments in major academic institutions receive considerable funding from drug companies.

Pharmaceutical companies extend their influence far into the world of research, and we have to question their ethics. The sad truth is, almost every big-name pharmaceutical company on the planet has been sued over **falsifying claims** for the efficacy of their drugs, or **hiding unflattering results** to trials, or **paying doctors back-handers** to push their products.

This is not 'conspiracy theory nonsense' or me trying to make my book more 'dramatic' or 'exciting', it's just the cold, hard, rather ugly truth. You can search online for press articles, and you will find I am telling the truth.

Where shall we start? How about **all** the world's largest drug companies; and how about we scan the news going back over the last 15 or 20 years? This lot should be enough to convince you that all is not well:

- **Pfizer. 2009.** *Pfizer To Pay $2.3 Billion In Biggest Fine Ever For Deceitful Drug Marketing.* See https://www.businessinsider.com/pfizer-to-pay-23-billion-in-biggest-fine-every-for-deceitful-advertising-2009-9
- **Pfizer. 2016.** *Pfizer fined record £84.2m for overcharging NHS.* See https://www.bbc.co.uk/news/business-38233852
- **Roche. 2012.** *Roche Failed To Report Thousands Of Drug Side Effects, Facing Fines.* See https://www.medicalnewstoday.com/articles/251891.php

- **Bayer. 2003.** *Bayer Agrees To Pay U.S. $257 Million In Drug Fraud.* See https://www.nytimes.com/2003/04/17/business/bayer-agrees-to-pay-us-257-million-in-drug-fraud.html
- **Bayer. 2008.** *Bayer fined $16.2M in price-fixing probe.* See https://www.fiercepharma.com/pharma/bayer-fined-16-2m-price-fixing-probe
- **Sanofi. 2017.** *Sanofi Pasteur Agrees to Pay $19.8 Million to Resolve Drug Overcharges to the Department of Veterans Affairs.* See https://www.justice.gov/opa/pr/sanofi-pasteur-agrees-pay-198-million-resolve-drug-overcharges-department-veterans-affairs
- **GlaxoSmithKline. 2012.** *GlaxoSmithKline fined $3bn after bribing doctors to increase drugs sales.* See https://www.theguardian.com/business/2012/jul/03/glaxosmithkline-fined-bribing-doctors-pharmaceuticals
- **GlaxoSmithKline.** Did they learn in 2012? Nope, back again in **2014.** *GlaxoSmithKline fined $490m by China for bribery.* See https://www.bbc.co.uk/news/business-29274822
- **Merck. 2016.** *Merck to pay $950 million for illegal marketing of Vioxx.* See https://edition.cnn.com/2011/11/22/health/merck-vioxx-fine/index.html
- **Johnson & Johnson. 2013.** *Johnson & Johnson fined $2.2bn to settle drug cases.* See https://www.bbc.co.uk/news/business-24811664
- **Johnson & Johnson. 2017.** *Johnson & Johnson faces $417m payout in latest talc case.* See https://www.bbc.co.uk/news/business-41003540
- **Novartis. 2017.** *South Korea fines Novartis $48 million for doctor kickbacks.* See http://www.fcpablog.com/blog/2017/4/28/south-korea-fines-novartis-48-million-for-doctor-kickbacks.html
- **Gilead. 2015.** *Gilead harmed patients by overpricing its drugs. But did it miscalculate?* See https://www.latimes.com/business/hiltzik/la-fi-mh-gilead-harmed-patients-20151201-column.html
- **Shire Pharmaceuticals. 2017.** *Shire fined $350 million in largest-ever bribery case of its kind.* See http://www.pharmafile.com/news/512245/shire-fined-350-million-largest-ever-bribery-case-its-kind
- **AbbVie. 2018.** *Court Rules AbbVie and Besins Healthcare Must Pay $448 Million in AndroGel Antitrust Case.* See

https://www.biospace.com/article/court-rules-abbvie-and-besins-healthcare-must-pay-448-million-in-androgel-antitrust-case/

- **AstraZeneca**. **2010.** *Pharmaceutical Giant AstraZeneca to Pay $520 Million for Off-label Drug Marketing.* See https://www.justice.gov/opa/pr/pharmaceutical-giant-astrazeneca-pay-520-million-label-drug-marketing

- **AstraZeneca**. **2016.** *AstraZeneca Agrees to Pay $5.5 Million to Settle Alleged Bribery Probe.* See https://www.wsj.com/articles/astrazeneca-agrees-to-pay-5-5-million-to-settle-alleged-bribery-probe-1472642361

- **AstraZeneca**. **2018.** *£20m 'secret payments' to plug drugs by AstraZeneca and Shire.* See https://www.thetimes.co.uk/article/20m-secret-payments-to-plug-drugs-by-astrazeneca-and-shire-ns2qrf7m2

- **Amgen. 2012.** *Amgen to pay $762 million, pleads guilty in marketing case.* See https://www.reuters.com/article/us-amgen-fine/amgen-to-pay-762-million-pleads-guilty-in-marketing-case-idUSBRE8BH0V620121218

- **Bristol-Myers Squibb. 2005.** *Bristol-Myers reaches $300 million settlement.* See http://www.nbcnews.com/id/8232237/ns/business-corporate_scandals/t/bristol-myers-settles-conspiracy-charge/#.XJ5j5pj7RPY

- **Bristol-Myers Squibb. 2007.** *Bristol-Myers Squibb to Pay More Than $515 Million to Resolve Allegations of Illegal Drug Marketing and Pricing.* See https://www.justice.gov/archive/opa/pr/2007/September/07_civ_782.html

- **Novo Nordisk. 2017.** *Novo Nordisk Settles U.S. Suit Over Victoza for $58.65 Million.* See https://www.bloomberg.com/news/articles/2017-09-05/u-s-sues-novo-nordisk-over-victoza-seeking-12-15-billion

- **Eli Lilly. 2009.** *Eli Lilly fined nearly $1.5B in drug marketing case.* See https://money.cnn.com/2009/01/15/news/companies/eli_lilly/

Seriously, I could do this all day.

Deceitful marketing claims. Hiding side effects, including increased cancer risks. Industry-wide bribery, especially doctor kickbacks. Falsified claims. Overpricing of drugs. Not exactly all sweetness and light, are they?

There are multiple examples to choose from for most of these companies. Some of these fines are for *billions*, not millions. The list above covers around $14.5bn in fines. Over the years, if the fines outweighed the profits, they would stop doing it. But clearly, the **cheating** is worth it. Even with the fines, these companies are making many billions in profits. This is big business. Very big business. And when big sums of money are involved, a lot of people tend to throw their ethics out of the window. Money talks.

Clearly, this is not just one or two isolated incidents. While I hate conspiracy theories, I have to say that there does seem to be some serious rot at the heart of the pharmaceutical industry. It seems clear to me, that if drug companies are funding research, there is likely some bias to that research, and the conclusions should not be completely trusted.

Does this mean that every employee of every drug company is a bad person? **Of course not.** Likely 95% or more of people worldwide employed in the pharmaceutical industry are *good people* with *good ethics* doing *good work*. But the few, highlighted in the media, spoil the big picture for the many. It's just a sad fact of life, virtually every big pharmaceutical company out there has been 'busted' and has paid up tens of millions or hundreds of millions in fines for their malpractice.

Medical journals

And finally, it's also a fact that many of the former editors[7] of the world's biggest and most well-respected scientific journals[8] openly lament the fact

---

[7] The BMJ Blog: *Richard Smith: Medical research—still a scandal.* (2014, Jan 31). Retrieved from https://blogs.bmj.com/bmj/2014/01/31/richard-smith-medical-research-still-a-scandal/

[8] The Ethical Nag blog: *NEJM editor: "No longer possible to believe much of clinical research published".* (2009, Nov 9). Retrieved from https://ethicalnag.org/2009/11/09/nejm-editor/

that a large proportion[9] of published research[10] is biased and unreliable[11]. I don't like this truth, I am not happy about this truth, but it is a truth. I could fill this book with hundreds of references, but the likelihood is that half of them would be useless, and if you wanted to, you could pick apart the design of the study, the methodology, the apparent bias, the conflicts of interest in funding (drug companies, food companies) or the authors credibility. I've spent 20 years reading and researching, and this is the conclusion I have reached. It pisses me off just as much as it pisses you off.

As the legendary John Ioannidis concluded in 2005, "Most Published Research Findings Are False." [12] In 2018, he demonstrated that the overwhelming majority of all research that has been done linking food, diet and nutrition, to health conditions and disease, is largely meaningless[13].

From the American Council on Science and Health, I quote[14]:

"Dr. Ioannidis bluntly states that nutrition epidemiology is in need of "radical reform." In a paragraph that perfectly captures the absurdity of the field, he writes:

"...eating 12 hazelnuts daily (1 oz) would prolong life by 12 years (ie, 1 year per hazelnut), drinking 3 cups of coffee daily would achieve a similar gain of 12 extra years, and eating a single mandarin orange daily (80 g) would add 5 years of life. Conversely, consuming 1 egg daily would reduce life expectancy by 6 years, and eating 2 slices of bacon (30 g) daily would shorten life by a decade, an effect worse than smoking. Could these results possibly be true?"

The answer to his rhetorical question is obviously no."

---

[9] *Editor In Chief Of World's Best Known Medical Journal: Half Of All The Literature Is False.* (2015. May 16). Retrieved from https://www.collective-evolution.com/2015/05/16/editor-in-chief-of-worlds-best-known-medical-journal-half-of-all-the-literature-is-false/

[10] Young S. N. (2009). Bias in the research literature and conflict of interest: an issue for publishers, editors, reviewers and authors, and it is not just about the money. *Journal of Psychiatry & Neuroscience* : JPN, 34(6), 412–417.

[11] Lexchin, J., & Light, D. W. (2006). Commercial influence and the content of medical journals. *BMJ (Clinical research ed.), 332*(7555), 1444–1447. doi:10.1136/bmj.332.7555.1444

[12] Ioannidis, JPA. Why Most Published Research Findings Are False. (2005) *PLoS Med 2*(8): e124. https://doi.org/10.1371/journal.pmed.0020124

[13] Ioannidis, JPA. The Challenge of Reforming Nutritional Epidemiologic Research. *JAMA. 2018;320*(10):969–970. doi:10.1001/jama.2018.11025

[14] *John Ioannidis Aims His Bazooka At Nutrition Science.* (2018. Aug 24). Retrieved from https://www.acsh.org/news/2018/08/24/john-ioannidis-aims-his-bazooka-nutrition-science-13357

You see how all this works? Do you need 47 pages of detailed references now? No, I don't think so. That's why I have kept references to a minimum, and just tagged them at the bottom of the relevant pages throughout the book, rather than building an entire chapter full of them at the back.

I am sorry, that took nine and a half pages to make my point, lengthy even for me. But now you know, why I have given references 'sparingly' throughout this book. This book is **my antidote to all that scientific confusion,** all those conflicts of interest, all that drug company meddling. Remember 'My Story' right back at the start - I read all the books, tried all the fad diets, read all the ridiculous claims in the newspapers, and after two decades of yo-yo dieting and feeling like shit, I was more confused than ever. In the end, I just defaulted to some *common-sense thinking*, tried things for myself, and kept track of what worked.

Over time, I learned to read books and research papers with a more critical eye, and I quit reading the nonsense in many newspapers, and the silly fad diet books, altogether. The end result of my own life experience and all my learning, is the **12 Core Principles** of *Mother Nature's Diet*. Given everything you have learned reading this book, I hope you will give the 12 Core Principles a try and see how they work for you.

Additional Reading

H aving covered all of that over the previous pages, in the interests of providing additional reading (and yes, a number of scientific journal references too) to those who are interested in learning more (or those wishing to check some additional sources to ensure that the material presented in this book is not just 'hocus-pocus' made up by some self-appointed wannabe-Internet-health-guru) over the next few pages I shall provide a few links and references to further reading that may interest you.

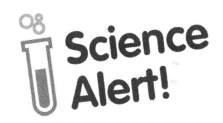

The economic burden of ill health due to diet, physical inactivity, smoking, alcohol and obesity in the UK: an update to 2006–07 NHS costs.[1]

From the Journal of Public Health. Quote *"...poor diet is a behavioural risk factor that has the highest impact on the budget of the NHS, followed by alcohol consumption, smoking and physical inactivity."*

Food and the responsibility deal: how the salt reduction strategy was derailed.[2]

From the BMJ. Quote *"The food we eat is now the biggest cause of death and ill health in the UK, owing to the large amounts of salt, saturated fat, and sugars added by the food industry."*

---

[1] Scarborough, P., et al., (2011). The economic burden of ill health due to diet, physical inactivity, smoking, alcohol and obesity in the UK: an update to 2006–07 NHS costs. *Journal of Public Health, Volume 33,* Issue 4, December 2011, Pages 527–535, https://doi.org/10.1093/pubmed/fdr033

[2] MacGregor G, A, et al. (2015). Food and the responsibility deal: how the salt reduction strategy was derailed *BMJ; 350* :h1936. doi: https://doi.org/10.1136/bmj.h1936

Quote *"Consuming too much energy from unnecessary sugar and fat causes obesity and type 2 diabetes, a rapidly increasing cause of death and disability."*

Quote *"Most of the foods that industry currently provides are very high in salt, fat, and sugars and are therefore more likely to cause cardiovascular disease and predispose to cancer than healthier alternatives. This is particularly true for people of low socioeconomic status as they tend to eat more cheap, processed foods."*

Quote *"If the food industry were made to produce healthier food, it would result in major* **reductions in both cardiovascular disease and cancer**, *as well as healthcare costs."*

What's Killing the World? High Blood Pressure, Poor Diet, Tobacco, Huge New Study Says.[3]

Quote *"A wide-ranging new global health study published in the medical journal The Lancet and funded by the Bill & Melinda Gates Foundation identifies the key risk factors for premature disease-related death worldwide: high blood pressure, poor diet, and tobacco use. In fact, poor diet alone is a risk factor for one in five global deaths, according to the research."*

Learn more, follow the **Global Burden of Disease.**[4]

GBD – Risk Factors Analysis.[5]

Quote *"In 2016 in 113 countries, the leading risk factor in terms of attributable DALYs was a metabolic risk factor."*

And that article goes on to point out that as we have reduced levels of smoking worldwide, reducing the preventable causes of NCDs, so metabolic factors have increased, offsetting those noticeable improvements. *In short – fewer folks are killing themselves with smoking, but more folks are doing it with poor diet and lack of exercise instead.*

---

[3] *What's Killing the World? High Blood Pressure, Poor Diet, Tobacco, Huge New Study Says.* (2017, Sept 15). Retrieved from http://fortune.com/2017/09/15/global-burden-of-disease-diet-tobacco-study/

[4] See more at: https://www.thelancet.com/gbd

[5] GBD 2016. Global, regional, and national comparative risk assessment of 84 behavioural, environmental and occupational, and metabolic risks or clusters of risks, 1990–2016: a systematic analysis for the Global Burden of Disease Study 2016. *The Lancet. Global Health Metrics, Vol. 390, Issue 10100*, P1345-14224. doi.org/10.1016/S0140-6736(17)32366-8

GBD again: **Poor diet is a factor in one in five deaths, global disease study reveals.**[6]

Quote *"Poor diet is a factor in one in five deaths around the world, according to the most comprehensive study ever carried out on the subject. Millions of people are eating the wrong sorts of food for good health."*

And finally, yet again from GBD: **Seven in 10 deaths fuelled by diet and lifestyle factors, study finds.**[7]

Britain's poor diet more deadly than its smoking habit as alcohol related deaths soar.[8]

Quote *"Cutting down on junk food diets, couch potato lifestyles, cigarettes and booze could make Britain one of the healthiest places to live in the world, while saving taxpayers billions on future NHS costs."*

That study[9] and **its reporting.**[10]

From Public Health England. Quote *"And even though there have been big falls in premature mortality, the top causes of early deaths in England and in each English region are still heart disease, stroke, lung cancer and chronic obstructive pulmonary disease, **which to a greater or lesser extent, are attributable to preventable risk factors.**"* - Professor John Newton, Chief Knowledge Officer, Public Health England

---

[6] *Poor diet is a factor in one in five deaths, global disease study reveals.* (2017, Sept 14). Retrieved from https://www.theguardian.com/society/2017/sep/14/poor-diet-is-a-factor-in-one-in-five-deaths-global-disease-study-reveals

[7] *Seven in 10 deaths fuelled by diet and lifestyle factors, study finds.* (2016, Oct 6). Retrieved from https://www.telegraph.co.uk/news/2016/10/06/seven-in-ten-deaths-fuelled-by-diet-and-lifestyle-factors-study/

[8] *Britain's poor diet more deadly than its smoking habit as alcohol related deaths soar.* (2015, Sept 15). Retrieved from https://www.telegraph.co.uk/news/health/news/11865074/Britains-poor-diet-more-deadly-than-its-smoking-habit-as-alcohol-related-deaths-soar.html

[9] GBD 2013. Changes in health in England, with analysis by English regions and areas of deprivation, 1990–2013: a systematic analysis for the Global Burden of Disease Study 2013. *The Lancet. Vol. 386,* Issue 10100, P2257-2274. https://doi.org/10.1016/S0140-6736(15)00195-6

[10] Public Health England. (2015, September 15). *England has the potential to have the lowest disease burden in the world.* Retrieved from https://www.gov.uk/government/news/england-has-the-potential-to-have-the-lowest-disease-burden-in-the-world

The burden of food related ill health in the UK.[11]

Quote *"The burden of food related ill health measured in terms of mortality and morbidity is similar to that attributable to smoking. The cost to the NHS is twice the amount attributable to car, train, and other accidents, and more than twice that attributable to smoking. The vast majority of the burden is attributable to unhealthy diets..."*

Poor diet 'biggest contributor to early deaths across the world'.[12]

Quote *"High blood pressure linked to bad diet contributed to most deaths, while smoking and air pollution were also high-ranking risk factors, study finds."*

Actual causes of death in the United States.[13]

Quote [abbreviated] *"The most prominent contributors to mortality in the United States in 1990 were tobacco...diet and activity patterns...alcohol..."* [And other factors] And *"Approximately half of all deaths that occurred in 1990 could be attributed to the factors identified."*

The combined effects of healthy lifestyle behaviours on all-cause mortality: a systematic review and meta-analysis.[14]

Quote *"A combination of at least four healthy lifestyle factors is associated with a reduction of the all-cause mortality risk by 66%."* In plain English - adhering to healthy lifestyle advice (such as in this book) reduces your risk of an early death by two thirds.

Healthy living is the best revenge: findings from the European Prospective Investigation Into Cancer and Nutrition-Potsdam study.[15]

---

[11] Rayner M, Scarborough P. (2005) The burden of food related ill health in the UK. *Journal of Epidemiology & Community Health* 2005;59:1054-1057.

[12] *Poor diet 'biggest contributor to early deaths across the world'.* (2015, Sept 11). Retrieved from https://www.theguardian.com/society/2015/sep/11/poor-diet-biggest-contributor-early-deaths-world-study

[13] McGinnis, J.M, Foege, W.H. (1993). Actual causes of death in the United States. *JAMA. 1993* Nov 10;270(18):2207-12. Retrieved from https://www.ncbi.nlm.nih.gov/pubmed/?term=8411605

[14] Loef, M., & Walach, H. (2012). The combined effects of healthy lifestyle behaviors on all cause mortality: a systematic review and meta-analysis. *Preventive Medicine, 2012* Sep;55(3):163-70. doi: 10.1016/j.ypmed.2012.06.017

[15] Ford, E.S., Bergmann, M.M., et al. (2009). Healthy living is the best revenge: findings from the European Prospective Investigation Into Cancer and Nutrition-Potsdam study. *Archives of Internal Medicine, 2009* Aug 10;169(15):1355-62. doi: 10.1001/archinternmed.2009.237

Diabetes and modifiable risk factors for cardiovascular disease: the prospective Million Women Study.[16]

Interesting quote *"Non-smoking women with diabetes who were not overweight or inactive still had threefold increased rate for coronary disease or stroke compared with women without diabetes."* I have said it before and it remains worthy or repeating – slim people die too. Non-smoking, not obese, and not sedentary/inactive, but with metabolic disease (type-2 diabetes) these women were still three times more likely to develop heart disease. If you eat a lot of sugar and you think you are 'getting away with it' because you are active and not overweight, think again. You might not be getting away with it after all.

Intensive Lifestyle Changes for Reversal of Coronary Heart Disease.[17]

Food consumption and the actual statistics of cardiovascular diseases: an epidemiological comparison of 42 European countries.[18]

Quote *"Our results do not support the association between CVDs and saturated fat, which is still contained in official dietary guidelines. Instead, they agree with data accumulated from recent studies that link CVD risk with the high glycaemic index/load of carbohydrate-based diets. In the absence of any scientific evidence connecting saturated fat with CVDs, these findings show that current dietary recommendations regarding CVDs should be seriously reconsidered."*

Chronic Diseases: The Leading Causes of Death and Disability in the United States.[19]

------

[16] Spencer, E.A., Pirie, K.L., et al. (2008). Diabetes and modifiable risk factors for cardiovascular disease: the prospective Million Women Study. European Journal of Epidemiology, 2008;23(12):793-9. doi: 10.1007/s10654-008-9298-3

[17] Ornish D, Scherwitz LW, Billings JH, et al. Intensive Lifestyle Changes for Reversal of Coronary Heart Disease. *JAMA. 1998*;280(23):2001–2007. doi:10.1001/jama.280.23.2001

[18] Grasgruber, P., Sebera, M., Hrazdira, E., Hrebickova, S., & Cacek, J. (2016). Food consumption and the actual statistics of cardiovascular diseases: an epidemiological comparison of 42 European countries. *Food & Nutrition Research, 60,* 31694. doi:10.3402/fnr.v60.31694

[19] U.S. National Center for Chronic Disease Prevention and Health Promotion. (2019). *Chronic Diseases in America.* Retrieved from https://www.cdc.gov/chronicdisease/resources/infographic/chronic-diseases.htm

Industry sponsorship and research outcome.[20]

Lifestyle and 15-year survival free of heart attack, stroke, and diabetes in middle-aged British men.[21]

Quote *"Modifiable lifestyles (smoking, physical activity, and BMI) in middle-aged men play an important role in long-term survival free of cardiovascular disease and diabetes. These findings should provide encouragement for public health promotion directed toward middle-aged men."*

Interesting reading: **The sun goes down on Vitamin D: why I changed my mind about this celebrated supplement.**[22]

And an interesting quote *"...massive analyses combining 27 studies on half a million people concluded that taking vitamin and mineral supplements regularly failed to prevent cancer or heart disease."*

Associations of fats and carbohydrate intake with cardiovascular disease and mortality in 18 countries from five continents (PURE): a prospective cohort study.[23]

Quote: *"High carbohydrate intake was associated with higher risk of total mortality, whereas total fat and individual types of fat were related to lower total mortality. Total fat and types of fat were not associated with cardiovascular disease, myocardial infarction, or cardiovascular disease mortality, whereas saturated fat had an inverse association with stroke. Global dietary guidelines should be reconsidered in light of these findings."*

---

[20] Lundh, A., Lexchin, J., Mintzes, B., Schroll, JB., Bero, L. *Industry sponsorship and research outcome.* Cochrane Database of Systematic Reviews 2017, Issue 2. Art. No.: MR000033. DOI: 10.1002/14651858.MR000033.pub3

[21] Wannamethee, S.G., Shaper, A.G., Walker, M., Ebrahim, S.. Lifestyle and 15-Year Survival Free of Heart Attack, Stroke, and Diabetes in Middle-aged British Men. *Archives of Internal Medicine. 1998;158*(22):2433–2440. doi:10-1001/pubs.Arch Intern Med.-ISSN-0003-9926-158-22-ioi80063

[22] *The Conversation: The sun goes down on Vitamin D: why I changed my mind about this celebrated supplement.* (2016, Jan 6). Retrieved from https://theconversation.com/the-sun-goes-down-on-vitamin-d-why-i-changed-my-mind-about-this-celebrated-supplement-52725

[23] Dehghan, M., Mente, A., et al. (2017, Nov 4). Associations of fats and carbohydrate intake with cardiovascular disease and mortality in 18 countries from five continents (PURE): a prospective cohort study. *The Lancet, Vol.390*, Iss 10107, P2050-2062. doi: https://doi.org/10.1016/S0140-6736(17)32252-3

Antioxidant supplements for prevention of mortality in healthy participants and patients with various diseases.[24]

Quote to note *"We found no evidence to support antioxidant supplements for primary or secondary prevention. Beta-carotene and vitamin E seem to increase mortality, and so may higher doses of vitamin A. Antioxidant supplements need to be considered as medicinal products and should undergo sufficient evaluation before marketing."*

Effects of Dietary Composition on Energy Expenditure During Weight-Loss Maintenance.[25]

Omega-3 Fatty Acids EPA and DHA: Health Benefits Throughout Life.[26]

6 million adults do not do a monthly brisk 10-minute walk.[27]

Shameful quote *"Over 6.3 million adults aged 40 to 60 do not achieve 10 minutes of continuous brisk walking over the course of a month and are missing out on important health benefits, according to [the] Public Health England..."* That is truly a woeful state of affairs here in the UK. I'm not one for supporting and kind of 'fat shaming' talk, but honestly, if 41% of British adults, between age 40 and 60, can't even get out and manage one brisk 10-minute walk per month, then we have to call it what it is - downright laziness. You can blame it on busy lifestyles, obesogenic environments, the rise of car culture, but these are excuses for laziness. Anyone can find a way to squeeze in a brisk walk once per week, anyone.

And quote *"...people in the UK are 20% less active now than they were in the 1960s and on average walk 15 miles less a year than 2 decades ago. The*

---

[24] Bjelakovic, G., Nikolova, D., et al. (2012) Antioxidant supplements for prevention of mortality in healthy participants and patients with various diseases. *Cochrane Database of Systematic Reviews 2012, Issue 3*. Art. No.: CD007176. DOI: 10.1002/14651858.CD007176.pub2

[25] Ebbeling, C.B., Swain, J.F., et al. (2012) Effects of Dietary Composition on Energy Expenditure During Weight-Loss Maintenance. *JAMA. 2012;307*(24):2627–2634. doi:10.1001/jama.2012.6607

[26] Swanson, D., Block, R., Mousa, S.A. (2012) Omega-3 Fatty Acids EPA and DHA: Health Benefits Throughout Life. *Advances in Nutrition, Volume 3,* Issue 1, January 2012, Pages 1–7, https://doi.org/10.3945/an.111.000893

[27] Public Health England. (2017, August 24). *6 million adults do not do a monthly brisk 10 minute walk.* Retrieved from https://www.gov.uk/government/news/6-million-adults-do-not-do-a-monthly-brisk-10-minute-walk

sedentary nature of modern, busy lives makes it difficult for many to find the time for enough exercise to benefit their health."

The recommendations are there: **Everybody active, every day: a framework to embed physical activity into daily life.**[28] But the people are not following them.

And from BHF: **Physical Activity Statistics 2015.**[29]

OK. Enough already. I could go on and on with references, links to papers, suggested further reading, but as explained previously, I don't see the point. Frankly, anyone with the time, experience in research, and inclination to do so, could go over every reference I have provided in the last few pages, and the dozens of other references provided throughout this book, and accuse me of cherry-picking data that supports my claims. I guess we are all subject to some confirmation bias. They could probably find contrary data to refute, rubbish or disprove that which I have shared, and an equal number of other references and links claiming a near-polar-opposite position. **Such is the world of academic research in the information age.**

In the end, dear reader, it comes down to you. You can choose to believe what I have presented in this book, or you can cast me aside and seek other sources of diet and lifestyle advice. It is entirely up to you. I would challenge you to 'suck it and see', to 'run it up the flagpole and see how it flies'. Try going just **90 days of your life** living by the 12 Core Principles of *Mother Nature's Diet* and see if what's in this book works for you. If 90 days sounds like too much, try following the 28-Day Plan, and see if just four weeks is enough to feel some of the benefits, and I think you'll be pleasantly surprised.

Learning more

This book is just an introduction to *Mother Nature's Diet* and the 12 Core Principles. If you would like to learn more, please visit our site at

---

[28] See: *Everybody active, every day: framework for physical activity.* From https://www.gov.uk/government/publications/everybody-active-every-day-a-framework-to-embed-physical-activity-into-daily-life

[29] See: *Physical Activity Statistics 2015.* From https://www.bhf.org.uk/informationsupport/publications/statistics/physical-activity-statistics-2015

www.MotherNaturesDiet.com and check out the free resources there, and follow my blog at www.MotherNaturesDiet.me.

Now you've read this book, if you are interested in going further with *Mother Nature's Diet*, you'll find everything you need on our site. Perhaps you would like to attend my very popular 1-day seminar, or our 3-day workshop, or maybe you'd like to come away with me for a week of healthy living and time in nature on one of our amazing mountain hiking retreats.

On the site you'll find more information about live events, trips, online video courses, further books that may interest you and information on how to join our monthly subscription-based membership community, MND Life!

If you have enjoyed this book, and if you have any feedback to share, I would love to hear from you, do please make contact through our website or find me or *Mother Nature's Diet* on social media.

You can use this page for your own notes.

The Last Word

For anyone who may feel inclined to dismiss *Mother Nature's Diet* and the 12 Core Principles as, "not scientific enough" or "too obvious" or "just a load of common sense really" (honestly, I actually take that as a compliment, I mean really, that's the goal here folks). Or for anyone who thinks quitting sugar and booze and junk food is "just too hard" or "a draconian lifestyle" or "too hardcore for normal people" then I'm going to ask those people for a **realistic viable alternative**. In fact, I won't take or respond to any such criticism unless you come offering a reasonable alternative way forward for the population of this wonderful country.

What I am trying to say is this: **If you are dismissing my solution, what solution do you offer instead, that can actually be promoted to a broad, nationwide audience with some realistic chance of acceptance and adherence?**

Let's be honest, the current mainstream approach is not working. Right? The government Eatwell Guide is not working; 5-a-day is not working (two thirds of the population don't do it); the food pyramid idea (in other countries) is not working; 'drink in moderation' is not working; 'everything in moderation' is not working; "enjoy a little of what you fancy" is not working; the 'diet industry' is not working; calorie counting is not working; the vast profusion of supplements, protein powders and vitamin pills are not working.

These 'solutions' have been around us for the last 20 years and yet over the same time period, things are just getting worse. Obesity on the rise. Type-2 diabetes on the rise. Autoimmune conditions on the rise. Mental health problems on the rise. I could go on. The point is, since the current mainstream health/diet/nutrition paradigm was introduced across the UK circa 1980, these key metrics we use to measure public health have not moved in the right direction. There have been amazing advances in surgical procedures, improvements in clinical diagnosis, improvements in drug treatments, nursing, early detection, smoking cessation, and more besides, all of which help extend life expectancy. However, these improvements are set off against a backdrop of increasing BMI and declining health and fitness among youth and younger (working age) adults.

323

In plain English: as fast as we are getting better at keeping sick, old folks alive for longer, we are getting worse at keeping fit young working-age adults, well, fit and young and working!

The increases in obesity, childhood obesity (in 2017 the Health Secretary described childhood obesity as "a national emergency" and many other health experts echo that statement [1]), type-2 diabetes, autoimmune conditions and reported mental health problems are all major causes for concern in UK public health.

So, before anyone dismisses *Mother Nature's Diet* because it's not written by a PhD in biochemistry, or a neurosurgeon with 40 years' experience, or a leading figure in Public Health England, kindly note that I offer a sensible, sustainable, affordable, enjoyable lifestyle, it's better for your health, the land, farmers, animal welfare, the environment and the future - but it will take some effort on your part, and it may incur either some extra work or a little additional expense. A small price to pay.

But if anyone is tempted to suggest this is too hard, or not realistic, then don't put my ideas down unless you can answer the question: "what better option do you offer?"

Public health in the UK faces some serious challenges. We've been called *"the fat man of Europe"* by the OECD[2], we drink too much and take far too little exercise. Our school report would definitely say "Could do much better."

In this book, you have learned that **you have more choice than you know.** There is a **sliding scale**, for your energy levels, your ability to resist ill health, your ability to resist the signs of ageing, and you can determine 50% to 75% of the story by your own free **choices.**

Now it's over to you. Time for you to take action. For many people, this is the lifestyle solution we need in a country struggling with chronic health challenges. I suggest you…

…just start.

---

[1] Mayor, S. (2016) Over a third of children aged 10-11 in England are overweight or obese. *BMJ 2016*; 355 :i5948. See
https://www.bmj.com/content/355/bmj.i5948.full
[2] *Britain is the fat man of Europe with 63 per cent of UK adults overweight.* (2017, Nov 11). Retrieved from
https://www.thetimes.co.uk/article/britain-is-the-fat-man-of-europe-as-obesity-doubles-in-two-decades-b5vx0nvsx

Acknowledgements

A FEW WORDS OF THANKS AND APPRECIATION

Without considerable help, guidance and encouragement, I doubt any book would ever actually get written. This book is no exception. There are many to whom I owe a debt of thanks.

I am grateful to life, for teaching me everything in this book, via a rather long and arduous journey, which involved quite a lot of beer, no small quantity of peanut butter sandwiches, and a couple of fairly painful butt-kickings along the way. Cheers for that. I'm also truly grateful to everyone and everything in my life that ever made me feel like shit, held me back, and said I couldn't do it. Thanks for making me the most driven, tenacious, truth-seeking realist on the block.

To my mum, as she rests peacefully, I'm grateful that she gave me my hard work ethic. And I'm grateful for all the good health habits she tried so hard to teach me, and I'm sorry it took me about 25 years to finally actually stick to them. To my brilliant sister, Lisa, for her creativity and loving stewardship of my beautiful branding. Her designs make me look like a grown up and for that I am eternally grateful. To my wife Steph, and our wonderful children, for their patience with me over the years as I learned what needed to be written in this book, and for her eagle-eyed editorial assistance under pressure. Our kids would probably prefer a dad who loves pizza and computer games, but they are young, teenagers, and I hope that as the years pass, they come to benefit from my nagging and our home-grown fruits and vegetables.

To my immeasurably wise and dear friend Dawn, who gives me far more encouragement, guidance and help than I ever adequately thank her for, I truly owe her so much. To my diverse, interesting and crazy friends Johnny, Bill, Stu, Shan, Trish, Sophie, Peter, Gary, Dave, Al and 'Team Lucky', for the nuggets of wisdom, the inspiration, and the carefully considered push in the right direction that they have all shared with me and which are all reflected in some way in this book. To my good friend Steven V. Mitchell for challenging me to change how I think about alcohol. Best. Thing. Ever.

I am grateful to Tony Robbins for being the catalyst, for challenging me to make a proper decision about who I wanted to be. Life really has never been the same again. I am both grateful for and influenced by, the writing and broadcasting of Robb Wolf, Mark Sisson, Lierre Keith, Dr Loren Cordain, Dr Rhonda Patrick, Richard Manning, Will Allen, Joel Salatin, Allan Savory, Dr Ben Goldacre, Dr Malcolm Kendrick, Dr Aseem Malhotra, Dr Rangan Chatterjee, Michael Pollan, Raj Patel, Dr Jason Fung, Patrick Holden, Dr Aseem Malhotra, Dr Shan Hussain, Dan Buettner, Alex Viada, Zoe Harcombe, Lord Nicholas Stern, Dean Karnazes, Larry Winget, Stephen Oppenheimer, Weston A. Price, Richard Wrangham, Charles Darwin and dear Dr Bruce Ames.

To my beloved MND Members, I am so completely indebted to you all, for your ceaseless patience, encouragement and kindness. I do what I do, for you, and I can only do what I do, thanks to you. You are my reason. To Michelle, Jason, Jane, Rachel, Jay, Jenny, Cassie, Lucy, Kat, Peter, Angie, Jacquie, Kerrie, Karen, Tim, Jacqui, Jamie, Kimmie, Sarah, Craig, Liz, Ralph and many others, you are the ones crazy enough to believe in me from the start. Your unending support, contributions to our community and enthusiasm for my work have enabled me to keep going, to get this book written, and for that I am so very thankful. *Mother Nature's Diet* is for all you guys, and I remain humbly in your service.

And last, but very definitely not least, I am eternally thankful to Mother Nature, for the sheer wonder and spectacle of life on Earth, in all its glorious and amazing beauty and complexity. If Earth were the size of an apple, the thin strip where all life exists, the soil, the oceans, and the atmosphere, is thinner than the apple's skin. If Earth were a beach ball, spray painted blue, all life as we know it exists in a layer thinner than that layer of spray paint. While facts like that continue to blow my mind daily, I will continue to be forever in awe of the wonderful, beautiful and quite fragile natural world that surrounds us. I remain committed to learning about, respecting and nurturing our environment for many years to come.

Legal Medical Disclaimer

The information and opinions provided in this document are designed for educational purposes only, and should not be taken as a substitute for medical advice or professional care. You should always consult with your doctor if you have any concerns about your health or any specific condition, treatment or if you plan to make any change to your diet or exercise routine. Do not use the information in this document to diagnose or treat any health problems or illnesses without consulting a licenced doctor.

No warranties or representations are made as to the accuracy of the information that appears in this document or at our web sites at www.MotherNaturesDiet.com and www.MotherNaturesDiet.me or other sites that may be linked from this document. If you click on links and visit websites from this document, you do so at your own risk. Any decision about your health or medical care based solely on information obtained from a commercial book, or from the Internet could be dangerous. Please consult a doctor with any questions or concerns you might have regarding your health. The author of this document cannot answer direct, personal medical queries, and cannot be held responsible for your health outcomes.

We hope that you will find information in this document of interest, but no responsibility of any nature whatsoever is accepted for any information contained in these pages. You use this information at your own risk. *Mother Nature's Diet* and MND Health Ltd are in no way liable for any use or misuse of any information obtained from this document or from our websites.

Printed in Great Britain
by Amazon

60181562R00199